Cognitive Fitness

The Psychology of Pain, Pleasure, and Purpose

D1173428

COGNITIVE FITNESS

PAIN IS INEVITABLE

HOW TO ALLEVIATE IT AND USE IT TO YOUR ADVANTAGE

ANIL RAJPUT

First published in Australia in 2019

Printed in India by Thomson Press India Ltd, New Delhi

ISBN 978-0-6485658-8-8

To all those people,
known and unknown, living and dead,
who suffered voluntarily
so that we can suffer less.

CONTENTS

INTRODUCTION

Hedonic motivation, which is to experience pleasure and avoid pain, is probably the highest level of abstraction that we can extract from a diverse range of human thought and behavior, and it seems to have unparalleled control over our lives. This abstraction may seem like an oversimplification, but no one consciously wants to suffer, and there is no other fundamental motivating force that unites us all, after a motivation for survival.

Compelled by the intrinsic hedonic motivation, we embark on a lifelong pursuit of happiness while hoping for a minimal amount of misery; however, most of us find it hard to experience enough happiness in life, and others, in search of ever-elusive happiness, feel infernal pain instead.

When happiness seems beyond the horizon, and when pain is all that is left in life, some keep living with the soul-crushing pain while others look to substance abuse for relief from the relentless discomforts, without realizing that pain can be alleviated and authentic happiness can be found with cognitive fitness.

Whether from excruciating emotional pain or from daily stress, you suffer more or less obviously. But what is not so obvious is that your health and prosperity are also affected when you are burdened by the pathological baggage of pain or chronic stress.

The onset of major medical conditions is virtually guaranteed when the stressors in your life keep startling you or when suffering has become a part of your life; and negative emotional states of mind are poisonous for your higher executive cognitive functions, which you need for success in the modern world.

Both suffering and stress are unwanted; however, coping with them to experience maximal happiness is not as easy as you think, and your pursuit of happiness or prevention of pain can reverse its course comfortably. Hedonic motivation appears to be deceptively simple, but it is too convoluted and perplexing to let contentment flourish; and pain sneaks quietly and easily into life.

The story seems incomplete and puzzling.

Pain and pleasure are an integral part of human life, and survival still seems to be the supreme goal of life; however, other life forms appear to exist without the sophisticated positive and negative emotions of the human brain. What purpose pain and pleasure serve for humans is an interesting question, and it raises several other questions.

If pain and pleasure are required for human life, why can contentment not be found comfortably, and why is pain more prevalent than pleasure? Why is happiness usually fleeting, and why can getting rid of pathological pain be extremely complicated and difficult? Why is the absence of any authentic pain not enough for happiness, and why is the pursuit of happiness alone usually futile?

If pain is unavoidable in life, is there anything we can do to alleviate it? More importantly, can we use the inevitable pain to our advantage?

This book not only tries to answer these puzzling questions (primarily with the help of psychology and neuroscience) but also presents practical strategies for you to experience continual happiness, within the bounds of possibility.

The psychology of cognition (thinking and other mental processes), emotion (pain and pleasure), action (behavior), perception, and imagination helps us to understand their association with the underlying mysterious motivations, which must be unraveled to alleviate suffering (or stress, anxiety, boredom, nihilism) and to advance happiness.

The human brain is the most complex entity known to itself, and the ability to use it advantageously is not always straightforward. Like any other complex system, the nervous system also has its limits. Unlike other man-made or natural systems, it also has intelligence, which is imperfect; and this fact makes all the difference.

Intelligence is marvelous, but the limits of our nervous system make it imperfect. Intelligence can help in your struggle for survival, but its imperfections can make you suffer more than that is destined for you.

Human intelligence has created magnificent things, but neurologically healthy people can also die by suicide because of the flaws in the cognitive and emotional elements of the human intellect and we will discuss several weaknesses of the human brain that can easily lead to mental disorders, and probably suicide in many cases.

In general, no other living thing seems to suffer or die by suicide like humans, and other life forms do not have advanced human intelligence. This fact makes a mockery of the practical utility of the human brain and its intellect. Suicide can be the worst case of the limitations that human intelligence places on our healthy mental function; however, in usual circumstances, human intelligence (and imagination) can easily introduce additional psychological pain in life, even without any apparent internal or external reason.

Psychology and neuroscience (and other fields) shed some light on the perfections and imperfections of the human brain and its intelligence. With this wisdom, and by keeping the weaknesses of your brain under control, you can use its strengths to endure inevitable pain and, surprisingly, use the pain to flourish.

In this book, some fundamental psychological and neurological facts, and a few cognitive strategies on the basis of those facts, are introduced (these strategies can become cognitive skills with enough practice); and such wisdom and cognitive strengths are part of your cognitive fitness.

The book not only tries to deal with the sheer complexity of the human brain but also of the external social and objective world and outlines the most critical knowledge and strategies in seven chapters.

Chapter 1 introduces the reason for pain, pleasure, and purpose and the complexity of the individual, social, and natural aspects of life. Chapter 2 discusses how a bounded brain deals with infinite information, the inevitability of illusions and ignorance, our ability to ignore our ignorance, the positive and negative aspects of the brain and illusions, and a few fundamental illusions of visual perception, cognition, and emotion. Chapter 3 summarizes the psychology of pain and pleasure, the deceptions of emotions, and the certainty and usability of pain and offers strategies for cognitive clarity. Chapter 4 explores why the human brain can be its own worst enemy and why it must be controlled by itself to flourish. Chapter 5 introduces the psychology of physical action, the efficiency of cognitive action, and the psychological significance of a subjective purpose or meaning of life, which allows us to explore the unknown, confront the chaos, and thrive. Chapter 6 discusses why focus or aim matters most and presents a well-known strategy to take control of it that also has numerous health benefits. Chapter 7 explains the importance of knowledge for our health, happiness, and success. It also highlights that we know almost nothing and that there is infinite potential in the cosmos; and as far as there are no biological deformities, life is always open for living.

Let's start with the reason for pain, pleasure, and purpose.

PAIN, PLEASURE, AND PURPOSE

Survival of the finite biological body and the mind in the infinite cosmos is the primary goal of life, and for us, in general, it is facilitated by the emotional feedback of the futility and utility of our thought (cognition) and behavior (action in space-time or simulation in mind).

Because survival is usually disguised behind emotional feedback, in the form of pain and pleasure, hedonic motivation appears to be the primary generalization, which can be inferred from collective human thought and behavior.

The feedback mechanism of pain and pleasure helps you to survive, but such feedback can be fundamentally flawed; and emotional feedback is not supposed to be the end goal of your life. Also, an emotion is not a solution, which is to think clearly and act again; and negative emotions often interfere negatively with your thoughts and behaviors.

These facts, associated with your hedonic motivation, are neither obvious nor easy to comprehend or exercise. Yet they are the primary source of avoidable suffering in your life. For example, substance abuse, consumption of junk food, overconfidence, and laziness may feel easy and pleasurable, but these positive emotions actually harm you bit by bit. Thinking, action, learning, being psychologically and physically fit, and wandering into the unknown may be effortful and painful at times, but they are the birthplace of all possibilities and potential. Moreover, the emotional prediction of pain and pleasure from things or events in the past and future is usually extremely overrated, but the suffering caused by the memory or imagination is real and when we face critical and complex challenges in life, continual negative emotions can easily make matters worse.

The inventory of inaccuracy, ambiguity, and usability of your emotions goes on and on. You need a lot of knowledge to be aware of the fantasies and fallacies of your own feelings.

The incomprehensible complexity of the human brain is bewildering; however, there is enough empirical evidence (which is introduced later in the book) that suggests that our emotions are subjected to errors or delusions and can be utterly unproductive or self-defeating and the end goal of life is survival, not positive or negative emotions.

Your brain is the most complex system known to itself, and the realization of its strengths and weaknesses, as well as its emotional framework, is the first step for dealing with hedonic motivation effectively.

You must take action to survive, and the negative emotional feedback that often ensues from your action is not the actual solution to the problem at hand. The solution is to pay attention, think clearly and critically, and act again with a correction in cognitions. If a negative emotion is not dead, after its life has run out as the feedback, the lingering pain can become pathological. You do not want pain in the first place; hence, accumulating it makes no sense. For this reason, the ability to detach yourself from your own negative emotions is the second step for dealing with the pitfalls of hedonic motivation.

You must prevent or override the illusory pain, which can easily account for a major part of pain in your life, and you must use any authentic pain as feedback to think, learn, and act again (for a better future, with peace and prosperity) or to come to a conclusion, if pain cannot be avoided.

Why pain (both illusory and real) is inevitable, and how you can use it for your health, happiness, and success, is discussed in detail later in the book. Ironically, if you know how to use pain effectively, it can be a blessing in disguise.

Your emotions can be confusing or irrational and a source of prolonged pain in your life, but your cognitions and perceptions are also subject to flaws, which further complicate the deceptive mechanism of hedonic motivation. A lot of objective information is needed to live a life that is free from decadence and unnecessary suffering caused by the errors of cognitions and perceptions; however, it is extremely difficult to come to this realization.

Fortunately, illusions of visual perceptions are obvious, and they provide irrefutable empirical evidence suggesting that subliminal activity in your head is subjected to errors (this subconscious activity is the source of your emotion, cognition, and perception). Therefore, we will discuss in detail the illusions and tricks of your visual perception. One such illusion of vision is introduced next, and more will follow in the next chapter.

Take a look at the two horizontal lines in figure 1, with fins attached to them, pointing in different directions. Which line appears longer?

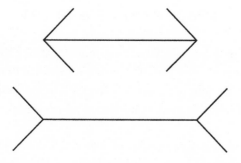

Figure 1

The length of the two lines may appear different, but a careful measurement will reveal that both are of the same length. If you have seen this image before, then you recognize it as the Müller-Lyer illusion. There are endless other optical illusions, and together they hold the absolute accuracy of the human brain as an object of ridicule.

Your brain is organized around vision, and almost half of your brain is dedicated to process visual perception, as opposed to the brains of most animals, which are organized around smell. If visual perception is not as authentic as it seems to be, the probability that all your cognitions and emotions are accurate, all the time, is zero. The inaccuracy of cognitions and emotions often causes misery (this is discussed more throughout the book).

An infinitely illusory dumb thought or emotion can force some people to take their own lives, and a cocktail of illusions is all that you need for a miserable life, without any apparent reason. Life can be brutal, and illusions of thoughts or emotions not only make it harder for you to manage the inevitable misery of life but also attach additional suffering to your existence. The most common illusions (objective and subjective) are discussed in this book, and you will feel liberated to know that most of your misery is likely to be illusory.

THE PURPOSE OF YOUR LIFE

In general, pain serves its purpose to motivate you to think and act and to solve problems. Ideally, pleasure is supposed to tell you that you are on the right path, but what happens when your survival is not on the line and there is no biological reason for the pain or pleasure?

While other living things seem to be satisfied with just survival, the behavior of the human brain is puzzling. If survival is not the current concern, and there is no justifiable reason for pain, the brain slowly starts to generate pain out of nothing and motivates you to do something more.

What you do beyond just survival is subjective to you, but the human brain is capable of known and unknown wonders, and something subliminal inside you encourages you to make use of the sleeping strengths of your brain and to think and act in ways that surpass simple survival.

The calling inside you, when you are not concerned about your survival, silently encourages you to find a purpose for your life and to transcend beyond simple survival. As you use your brain to its full extent, you can do your part to uplift your family, your community, and the collective life.

In general, despite the pain and perplexity in life, which paints a pessimist picture, you can almost always flourish. In addition to pain, there is realistic hope as well. You can always use pain to propel you toward your goal, which is the primary purpose of pain.

After a primary motivation to survive, striving for greatness is the secondary abstraction of collective human thought and behavior; however, it seems like a slumbering potential that needs to be awakened.

Hedonic motivation motivates you to survive, make your present pleasurable, and move toward a better future in the space-time; this motivation framework usually runs your life. Why motivation matters, and what having a purpose for your life can do for you, is discussed next.

The visual illusion shown in figure 1 tells you something startling. Your brain does not see the world and its objects in accurate or complete detail but as what it means, with motivation as a primary maneuver. This meaning can be inaccurate, but you would not be able to live without it.

Motivation guides your perception, cognition, emotion, and action; they all are part of one framework. With the help of visual perception, you act in the space-time with a motivation or goal. Your emotions (positive and negative) provide feedback of your action, and your cognitions can correct your subjective map of the objective world, according to the feedback.

Your intelligence, imagination, and the rest of your neural abilities are also part of the same motivation framework. In general, intelligence is your ability to find a solution to a complex problem, using other elements of the motivation framework; imagination is simulating the solution in your head, without acting out in the real world. Here a problem is what prevents you from reaching your goal, and without a motivation, there are no problems, just objective facts.

In evolution, intelligence and imagination seem to emerge from the motivation of survival; however, we can use these abilities to think abstractly about the infinite objective world and to observe the breathtaking beauty and mystery of the cosmos.

Even if there is no purpose or problem in your life, human intelligence and imagination are not supposed to make your life miserable in the present. Memory is where everything is stored, and it is also supposed to be on your side. However, intelligence, imagination, and memory are not always your friends, without any conscious and effortful oversight, something we will review in detail later.

To live in space and time, a motivation is needed to make sense (or find a meaning) of the limitless information available in the universe. Perceptions create an extremely simplified but meaningful version of the convoluted cosmos instantly and automatically, with probable errors. These errors of a limited nervous system are inevitable, as we have seen in figure 1, and the reason behind the errors is the utter complexity of the cosmos.

Visual perception is effortless and seems simple, but it is exceptionally complicated, and this complexity became apparent in the scientific world with the advent of research into artificial intelligence (AI). Scientists realized that there is infinite information at multiple levels—cellular, molecular, atomic, and subatomic, for example—and without a motivation to act (for some goal) in the space-time, AI software cannot focus on finite information at a particular scale in space.

Without a focus (or an aim), infinite information makes no sense to human or artificial intelligence, and both nervous systems and machines have limited memory and can focus on only a finite amount of information at a time.

The rise of robotics helped AI researchers to understand natural intelligence because a robot is supposed to act in space-time with an aim (motivation), and eventually the common link among intelligence, perception, aim, and action became noticeable. However, researchers are still struggling with the problem of perception (and action), and the most powerful supercomputers cannot perceive what you automatically perceive with your senses, without any conscious cognitive effort.

Millions of years of evolution seem to have designed our vision with survival as the primary purpose. Out of the infinite known and unknown, only finite information is perceived and assigned a meaning automatically, which helps you to act and to be alive as a mobile creature. For example, you see things that are food so that you can eat them, and you see predators so that you do not become food; you do not see atoms or subatomic particles in a fruit or in a predator.

You see a tiny part of the actual world so that you can think, act, and live; meaningful motivation is a must to function in the infinite cosmos. A meaning is assigned to the relevant information, as deemed fit by the brain, which may or may not be accurate or complete. Meaning or purpose in life is not always about accuracy because absolute accuracy is not possible with a limited brain, and motivation is all that matters. When your survival is taken care of, you can find a secondary motivation in the form of the purpose (or meaning) of your life, which not only makes sense to you but also gives you hope for a better future and lets you live in peace in the present.

Your brain can do wonderful things if you focus it on the finite in the infinite. Without an authentic long-term motivation, all the elements of your motivation framework are likely to make you suffer. For example, the purpose of positive and negative emotions is to give you the momentary feedback of your action in the moment. Action is supposed to be driven by a motivation, and your intellect can help you to think and solve problems as you move in the space-time toward your goal—or simulate the solutions in your head with imagination. Both positive and negative emotions are supposed to be fleeting feedback of your action or imagination, and a desire for only pleasure or the absence of any pain is in direct conflict with the biological reality. In general, such unrealistic desire is conducive to pain, not pleasure.

Also, without long-term motivation, your actions, cognitions, emotions, perceptions, intelligence, and imagination have no leadership; all can act randomly without any coherence whatsoever. Having a mind without a definite motivation is like being in a boat, where all the rowers are trying to take the boat in an arbitrary direction. In real life, without a motivation, you do not go anywhere, or you may easily go to the infernal world of suffering.

Pain is inevitable in life, but much of it can be brought under control with a long-term motivation. Without a motivation, most pain can easily be self-inflicted by the motivation framework. More on this is discussed later.

Taking control of your positive or negative states of mind from the inside; realizing that we know almost nothing; experiencing and exploring life to its fullest, without any assumptions or conclusions; and letting the force of life inside you flourish with complete openness are some good objective goals, whereas to suffer because of delusions of cognitions and emotions can be just a choice.

Without definite goals, some keep living with avoidable suffering, and some abuse substances for happiness. Several drugs artificially activate the same motivational or exploratory pleasure-generating neural circuits that well-defined goals for life can activate naturally. Drugs can boost happiness for a short period of time, but with dangerous side effects, whereas a long-term motivation can generate continual positive emotions, without any side effects. More on this is discussed throughout the book.

There is infinite information in this world, which can be interpreted in infinite ways, and there are infinite paths for you to tread. However, the ability of your brain to perceive, process, store, and retrieve information is limited. Out of the infinite known and unknown, your brain can deal only with the finite, which is guided by your purpose, and the rest is completely and constantly ignored. Your brain needs a primary aim to function properly in the vastness of the cosmos; without it, you may be lost in infinity.

Reliance on randomness, for an arbitrary motivation, is not a great strategy to deal with hedonic motivation, which is part of the higher motivation framework. You need a purpose for your life, which stays with you all along, and this strategy directs incredible strengths of your brain toward a manageable and meaningful finite to bring order to the chaos.

Finding a purpose for your life and moving toward it with courage completely changes the way your nervous system works, and we will discuss why this strategy is substantially superior to reacting to the arbitrary or transitory desires (with pleasure as an end goal) of hedonic motivation.

Your motivation framework is more powerful than you think, and it can make you suffer or thrive; it depends on your motivation. A purpose for your life can activate the sleeping strengths of your nervous system and bring your brain and your being into coherence. Your brain is equipped to do difficult things, but without a purpose, it may not let you live in peace.

It is always liberating to know that despite the inherent suffering of life, most of us can minimize suffering, feel good in the present, and eventually thrive. Alleviating suffering, feeling positive in the present, and moving forward toward greatness and hope are some of the recurrent themes of this book.

If you already have a purpose but find it difficult to attain, or if you had one but gave up after multiple failures, or if you are open to one but think you cannot attain it, cognitive fitness can help you and can put you on the right track.

NIHILISM

Being nihilistic is not the best way to live your life.

Science is the study of objective abstractions of the observable universe, and all the subjectivity must be stripped off for the scientific method. However, without a subjective moral hierarchy, you cannot decide which motivation must be preferred over infinite others.

Without a doubt, science has helped in the survival of the human race (with applied sciences: for example, engineering and medicine), but it has also given rise to the death of a subjective sense of life (and environmental pollution). When we know about the objectivity of the universe, subjective purpose may seem useless in the infinite objective cosmos. However, there are several problems with that line of thinking. A few are discussed next.

By definition, science cannot suggest the subjective purpose of your life because subjectivity is stripped in the first place. Observing the objectivity of the universe is fine, but you also have the mysterious and mystical ability to observe other objects. You are an observer, as well as a highly complex object, and both seem equally real.

Even those who believe that they know everything—and that life is futile and we are all just doomed objects—do not kill themselves because they value their lives, but they cannot comprehend it consciously. An action matters more than a thought, and the mismatch between cognition and action is puzzling.

Death, disease, disability, and suffering in life make a mockery of the assumption that we know everything. We are aware of a few principles of the known universe, but there is still an infinite amount to be learned. A little objective understanding of the world cannot conclude, as of now, that we know all or that we will be able to understand every single thing in the future.

Only the future can tell what it holds for humans, but as of now, we know almost nothing, and sometimes it is hard to separate nihilism from a naive narcissism.

We have formulated many fundamental facts of this universe—for example, gravitational and electromagnetic forces, subatomic particles and their properties, the speed of light, and the rest—but we do not know the source of those facts or what lies beyond.

Facts of science (and subjectivity) also seem to change over time and space. For example, classical (Newtonian) mechanics was considered complete once, but quantum mechanics changed that assumption, and the laws of physics change as the scale of space changes.

The laws of quantum mechanics (or of a black hole) are not the same as the laws of the scale of space that we inhabit. No one knows about all the laws that govern this universe and beyond or the mysterious laws that control the laws of this universe.

Subjective facts seem permanent also, but they may not stay the same with time or space. Your subjective interpretation of facts can change with the flick of a switch, as new facts emerge. For example, a betrayal can change your past and your understanding of yourself, others, and the world, and a success can change your future forever. What appears to be a subjective fact can become an illusion in a moment.

Empiricism (a belief that objective facts can be acquired through observation) makes the scientific method (using empirical evidence to find the facts) possible, but it cannot prove a theory (a hypothetical explanation of an aspect of the natural world) right because a hypothesis (a falsifiable prediction of a theory) can be falsified in a future experiment, even if it has not until now.

In the objective and rational scientific world, you can be proven wrong, not right, but to live a life, you must define moral right or wrong; the observer is where empiricism starts. Rationality alone is of no use without motivation, emotion, and the body of an observer.

From finite known facts of the universe, infinite facts emerge—and from them infinite interpretations—and you, as an observer, with limited neural resources, cannot focus on the infinite. Your subjective moral structure can guide you to focus on the finite, and without it, you are lost in the infinity and chaos.

You can understand some branches of science, such as physics, chemistry, and mathematics, by sitting in a room or experimenting in a lab, but to understand life, you must also understand its complicated history, which seems to span billions of years.

With a little understanding of some branches of science, many may conclude that life can also be understood by focusing on a few objective facts, but you also must have knowledge of several branches of humanities and social sciences (primarily philosophy and psychology) to be aware of the complexity of morality and subjectivity; and if there are no neurobiological imperfections, philosophy matters more than physics for a flourishing life.

A lot of death and suffering has brought us the relative peace of the modern world, for which we are usually not grateful. Our ancestors have tried to make sense of the world and have embedded the learned wisdom in philosophical stories and poems, using symbolism and archetype. The stories written and enhanced by the wise across several generations summarize the indispensable survival strategies and philosophies, which we ignore at our peril.

The great work and wisdom of our ancestors, abstracted into fictional or mythological stories, is seen as suspicious in the modern scientific world; meanwhile, watching movies or animation seems just fine.

The god in the archetypal stories is an archetypal hero who faces the suffering of life and does not become corrupt or weak; this is a similar role played by a usual hero in a modern movie. You embody the hero when you watch a movie, and the fiction makes sense to something deep inside you, just as the music, dance, or sport does.

It is the similar subliminal subjective philosophical sense in yourself that you need to function properly in life, even when it is hard for you to articulate it consciously.

The collective classic literature of humankind has incomprehensible depth, wisdom, and philosophical meaning, which is impossible to formulate on your own, just as you cannot invent all the science by yourself.

Nihilism is a thought that you know everything, inside and outside, and that the observer alive inside you does not matter. However, you do not have any direct access to the multiple layers of the subconscious and the mysterious unknown inside yourself, and you do not know exactly why some ideas make sense and others do not.

The idea to have a purpose in life may not make any sense to the objectivity and rationality domains, but subjectivity is a different domain, and a subjective purpose can transcend your life, which is beyond suffering and nihilism.

If we can ever know everything, that will be a sight to see, but until then, humility in our limitation is a better strategy. It does not mean that we do not seek more knowledge of the objective world and remain curious but that we also acknowledge our ignorance and arrogance.

It is hard to define what is real and what is not, and until the problem of integrating what is and what should be is solved, whatever makes your life and the collective life less miserable is probably the best definition of reality (biological reality), and you are free to use science as a tool for your survival.

Knowing that two plus two is four is not life. It is much more than that.

Harmony between objectivity and subjectivity is a good thing. Facts have no end; you cannot wait to live fully until all the facts are in. Even if they are available, you can focus on only one fact at a time, and you do not have enough time to go through them all. You have limited time on this earth, and wasting it in eternal confusion has no practical utility.

Not every problem can be solved, and not every question can be answered. A little humility in our limitations and gratitude for the gift of life can help us find a subjective meaning in life, without which life often struggles to flourish.

Nihilism leaves you with nothing in the face of suffering; however, people who believe that life has no purpose still act as if the life inside them matters. This mismatch between thought and action is paradoxical and puzzling.

Stating that there is only an objective world, from a subjective world, is always amusing.

COGNITIVE FITNESS

The universe is an extremely complex place, and your brain tries its best to hide the complexity of the cosmos from you; however, a betrayal, a crushed dream, hopelessness, a death or disability, or another anomaly can easily unveil the concealed complexity.

When chaos emerges from the underlying unknown, it disrupts the comfortable order in your life. As the terrifying unknown becomes the known, the illusion of simplicity withers away. To make matters worse, negative emotions are likely to overwhelm and degrade your ability to think clearly (to solve problems) when you need it the most.

Solving complex problems requires thinking at its best, and when many problems strike at once or accumulate over time, thinking can become increasingly useless or self-destructive. You may or may not be aware of the accuracy or utility of your thinking (and your emotions), and even if you are, controlling your mind (and emotions) can be like trying to control the air with your bare hands.

Life is difficult; ironically, it is also difficult in the absence of any real difficulty (which often leads to boredom), and illusions of thoughts and emotions can make you suffer even in the most serene situations. For all of us, solving problems in life, in the presence or absence of difficulty, is not as simple as it seems.

Both the living world and the brain are extremely complex, but the complexity is not always obvious. For example, eating food is easy in stable societies, but finding a partner or a job, starting a new business, managing stress, or thriving in life may not be easy for everyone in any society, and quitting smoking, overcoming alcohol addiction, stopping abuse of drugs or other substances, finding food in failed societies, and facing unusual pain in life is almost never easy.

When the problems of life do not go away, we can see they are convoluted, and with the realization of the multilayered complexity of the internal and external worlds, you can either solve them or, if they cannot be solved, come to a philosophical conclusion.

Overall, it is usually not easy to solve a complex problem without some knowledge of the complexity of the internal and external worlds and how they interact with each other. To understand this concept more completely, consider the complexity of a smartphone and your brain.

When you use an advanced mobile phone, it just works, but the complexity exists at multiple levels—subatomic, atomic, molecular, microelectronic, electrical, computation, communications, software, and artificial intelligence—and other technical aspects also play a role. Economic, social, and political factors contribute as well. All this complexity is hidden behind a simple user interface that you can interact with using your fingers and eyes.

A smartphone is not one system but a collection of highly complex systems working in coherence, and a tiny disturbance at any level is enough to bring the whole set of systems down. When your phone stops working, apart from trying a restart or the usual troubleshooting, there is nothing much that you can do.

A mobile phone represents the complexity of the objective scientific world; however, a working phone is also dependent on the social world. You can hardly study science in a society where crime and corruption are prevalent or where there is no social security and a scarcity of food.

Science explains what we already know about nature, but still there is infinite to be known, and we know only a little about biology. We can make a new mobile phone, or fix a broken one, with the help of science in a stable society, but the biology of the brain takes the complexity to a completely new level because we understand only a little about it (whereas we know and can learn everything about a mobile phone).

The complexity of a human brain puts that of a smartphone to shame. There are several known and unknown layers of both physical and abstract elements that structure and shape your brain (and the rest of the body), including atoms, molecules, genetics, cells, organs, physiological and psychological states, family, individuality, society, finance, politics, history, and so on. Problems in your life can be because of a minute disturbance at one or multiple layers, and unfortunately, it is not always obvious.

You may try to use your brain to solve a complex problem, but without the knowledge of complexity of the natural, social, familial, and individual attributes of your existence, your efforts may be unproductive. For example, a depression (or any other continual dysfunction or disturbance in cognition, emotion, and action) can be because of a natural imbalance of chemicals (neurotransmitter, hormone, vitamin, mineral, and the rest) or any other biological condition; difficulty or malevolence in your social environment; a broken family; a lack of experiences, knowledge, and skills; your cognitive and physical lifestyle; objective or subjective illusions of cognitions and emotions; or something else entirely.

Sometimes a simple test and a supplement can relieve the depression, and other times you must transform yourself mentally and physically, which can take months or years; and you cannot always control everything internally or externally. Whatever the case, it is not always easy to figure out the source of and solution to a depression—or any other convoluted problem.

Finding the root cause of a problem (if it is possible) to solve it (or come to a conclusion if it cannot be solved) is a superior strategy to doing nothing, blaming (yourself, your family, your community, or nature), or trying your luck with arbitrary solutions.

Awareness of the complexity can motivate you to acquire knowledge (by reading, experiencing new things, and learning), and knowledge can help you to pinpoint the problem, in the multiple layers of abstractions, or to comprehend and conclude that not every problem is solvable.

Knowledge can make you aware of how the convoluted elements of the motivation framework interact with one another and with the external, infinitely complicated world. Knowledge can also help you to explore the unknown (for opportunities and new information), conceptualize strategies, and develop cognitive skills.

To be known in this world is infinite, and infinite is unknown, and untapped unknown may be scary, but it is where the infinite potential is. You can explore the latent unknown voluntarily, or you can be forced to explore it by some adversity, or you may be lucky enough to live a relatively happy life, without much thinking or pain, at least as of now. But uncertainty is built into the fabric of space-time, and change is always lurking.

Whatever the case, advanced knowledge of the internal and external worlds, exploration of the unknown, and a few fundamental cognitive strategies and skills that make you competent and confident can prevent your downfall into the underworld and allow you to flourish.

Cognitive fitness is the high-level understanding of the complex aspects of several scientific and philosophical fields that make up the individual, familial, cultural, and natural elements of a human life. It is the development and continuation of a few indispensable cognitive skills through grueling cognitive workouts that promote cognitive fitness.

Cognitive fitness means having above-average knowledge of positive and negative aspects of the individual, family, social structure, and Mother Nature, and it means having the ability to use this knowledge to live a least miserable and thriving life, one that also makes a subjective sense to you.

Problems can exist in multiple dimensions, and focusing on only one thing in one area is not going to solve a complex problem. Awareness of both good and bad aspects of body and of mind, family, society, and the natural world can help you to succeed in what you are trying to achieve. A brief introduction to the positive and negative aspects of all four elements follows, and they are also discussed throughout the book.

Mother Nature gives us life, but it also rewards us with suffering, to a greater or lesser degree, in an unfair manner. Some are gifted with perfect genes and a thriving environment, and some come into this world with biological deformities in the most difficult places on the earth.

Nature is not fair, and all kinds of inequalities are built into nature. Some things are distributed normally, statistically speaking, and others are distributed randomly or selectively by nature. For example, most people have a working mind and body, but not all; and a huge success depends on randomness, along with the effective use of internal and external resources.

Similarly, a society has rules that restrict you; however, society also keeps you alive. Nature will kill you soon enough, if you are alone in the wilderness, without the several protective layers of society. A society where truth and trust are paramount provides a platform from which you can thrive, but it can never be perfect. You can have equality of opportunity in a healthy society (if you are gifted with a working mind and body by nature), but Mother Nature controls equality of outcome. No one knows how to solve this problem.

Similar to a society, a family (if you have one) supports you and restricts you. You have responsibilities in a family and your freedom is usually constrained, but without a family, life can become a living hell. Humans are social animals, and our brains are evolved to connect with other humans; an absence of such human connection is usually predictably miserable.

Finally, your brain is the most complicated structure known to humankind, and this book is primarily dedicated to exploring the positive and negative aspects of the human brain.

Premature death and suffering in the modern world can be caused by a lack of cognitive and physical fitness. Physical fitness undeniably helps, but if you are stressed, bored, depressed, anxious, or nihilistic most of the time, you need something superior to a physical workout, and physical fitness is a subset of cognitive fitness.

The story of life is identical for most of us. Life is usually good, an anomaly occurs, you go to hell, and you may or may not come out of it to feel good or hopeful again. Cognitive fitness prepares you in advance for cognitive and physical action to face changes and challenges head-on and to achieve greatness, and if you are already in trouble, it can rescue you from the deepest abyss.

INFORMATION AND ILLUSIONS

Perception facilitates our survival by creating a finite internal representation of the external world, which has infinite information; and our intelligence separates us from the rest of the living organisms. We share some primal emotions (fear and panic, for example), motions (find food and partner in the space, for instance), and motivations (to live and reproduce) with other animals. We also have uniquely human emotions, motions, and motivations as well as sophisticated cognitions and imagination.

Although each living cell has memory and intelligence that is still beyond our current scientific knowledge, neural circuits are the known source of human intelligence and other wonders of the human brain.

A neural circuit is a collection of neurons and neurotransmitters, among other things. Neurons are information-processing cells and neurotransmitters are molecules. Neural circuits are overwhelmingly complicated and fascinating, but there are not enough neurons for information-processing perfection, and each neuron has a limit.

The systematic or subjective imperfections of neural circuits give rise to illusions, where subjective reality differs from the objective or biological reality (which can be defined as whatever helps in collective survival, with the least amount of suffering). Although some of these illusions inflict no harm and actually help, others can be easily detrimental to your health, happiness, and success.

This chapter outlines how illusions of perception, cognition, and emotion emerge from the imperfect information processing of the neural circuits, and the enormous negative effect of the illusions (of thoughts and emotions) on your well-being is discussed throughout the book. We will also discuss strategies to administer and alleviate the miserable consequences that can be inflicted by the illusions.

VISUAL ILLUSIONS

We presented an example of optical illusion earlier, and we will now look at a few more. In figure 2, the color of the horizontal bar appears to fade out from right to left, but in reality, the shade of gray is exactly the same throughout the horizontal bar. The horizontal lines in figure 3 do not seem to be parallel to each other, but in reality, they are.

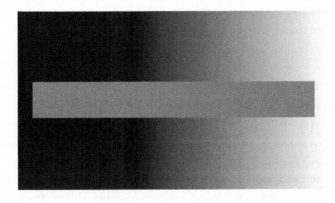

Figure 2
Contrast illusion

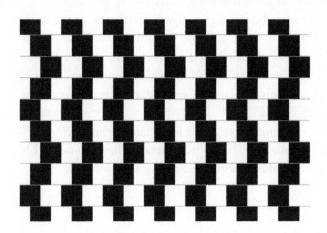

Figure 3
Café wall illusion

The illusions in figures 1, 2, and 3 seem to suggest that one part of your brain can distort objective information (when it is available), and the other part of your brain can detect the distortion.

Using your thinking, you can be aware of an illusion, but you cannot help but see the same distortion every time you look at the same picture. The best you can do is to know an illusory pattern (perceptual, emotional, or cognitive) in advance and bring this knowledge back into your awareness every time you perceive a similar pattern, taking corrective action if needed.

We will discuss the suffering that distortions of cognition and emotion can produce, and because awareness of the illusions of cognitions and emotions is not enough to stop them all the time, we will also discuss fundamental strategies that can prevent or minimize suffering, real or illusory.

Your brain can not only distort the available information, as we have seen in figures 1, 2, and 3, but also can create brand-new information when it is absent. To illustrate this, close your left eye and focus on the plus sign in figure 4 with your open eye. Keeping the book in front of your eye, bring the book closer to your nose. Keep your eye focused on the plus sign while remaining aware of the presence of the black circle. At some point, the black circle will disappear—only to appear again if you keep moving the book toward your face.

The disappearance of the black circle is an interesting illusion because your brain fills in information when it is unavailable. But why is the information missing in your visual field?

Figure 4
The filling-in illusion. Your brain can make the black dot disappear if it is at a specific distance from your eye.

The eye's lens (figure 5) bends the incoming light from an object and focuses it on the retina to form an upside-down image of that object. Photoreceptor cells (cones for color vision during the light and rods for black-and-white vision during the dark) in the retina convert visible light into neural impulses, which are transmitted to the brain by the optic nerve. The optic nerve leaves the retina through a hole called the blind spot. Because there are no photoreceptor cells at the blind spot, the brain does not receive any information about the part of the image formed at the blind spot.

When you bring the book closer to you, at a certain distance, the image of the black circle falls on the blind spot in your eye. Because your eye does not have sensory neurons at the blind spot, it cannot perceive the presence of the black dot. But instead of showing you nothing or some predefined color, your brain shows you the color that surrounds the blind spot. In figure 4, the space surrounding the black circle is white, and therefore your brain shows you a white color at the blind spot. Because you cannot differentiate a white circle in a white surrounding, the black circle disappears.

When you keep moving the book toward your nose, the image of the black circle falls out of the blind spot and you see the black circle again.

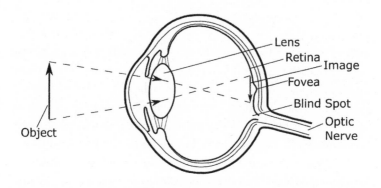

Figure 5
The human eye

Distortion and creation of information by the brain can invite trouble without any reason, and we will come back to both of these concepts later in the chapter. First, let's move on to the other imperfections of the brain.

Further to distortion and creation of information, what you see is extremely limited, which is obvious, because you cannot see an atom or the edge of the universe, if there is any. What you see, out of what you can see, depends on your motivation or focus; both of these factors also affect your well-being.

Your vision is clearest at a tiny part of your retina, called the fovea, which we can see in figure 5. There are around 120 million rods and six million cones in each of your eyes. The fovea has most of the cones, without any rods, and the rest of the cones are sparsely distributed across your retina. The resolution of a color image increases with the number of cones, hence your usual daytime visual resolution is highest at the fovea. During the night, the rest of the retina works better with rods.

The number of rods or cones in your eye is analogous to the number of pixels (usually referred to as a megapixel, which is one million pixels) in a digital camera.

Finding evidence of the high and low resolution of your eye, because of the distribution and number of rods and cones across your retina, is easy. Without moving your eyes or head, try to focus on the farthest object you can see, to the left or right, in your peripheral vision. You will notice that the visual perception of every object is blurred. However, if you move your eyes, head, or both toward the blurred object, at one point, the projected image of the object falls on the fovea, and you see it in high resolution.

Your peripheral vision is sensitive to movement in the environment, largely for the detection of predators.

It may not be obvious that the resolution of what you see at a given time varies, as you focus only on a part of it with highest clarity. You see only one little object, or a small part of a big object, with clarity, and there is an illusion of clarity for the rest of the image. When you move your eyes or head or both, the transition from low resolution to high resolution is automatic and smooth, as if you were seeing the whole image in high resolution all the time.

Your visual perception can work at full resolution for only a tiny object. This highest level of perceptual information is almost nothing when compared with the complete information available in the object at different levels of resolution. For example, there are billions of atoms in the smallest object that you can see, but you cannot see even one of those atoms.

Now, if you are cognitively loaded and your vision is focused on an object of interest only, you will not see other objects if their image does not fall on the fovea. Your vision is not only limited but also can be blind to what is right in front of you, if your focus is diverted even slightly.

Your sight is limited, and in general, you see what you focus on and what you expect to see. The implication of these factors is beyond imagination.

Researchers have conducted several studies in which people failed to notice the obvious (inattentional blindness) or a change (change blindness) in their environment, and the results were not surprising. After all, you see, smell, and hear so many things in each moment, but you can focus on only some part of it, and even that focus can be of no use if it is diverted.

For example, if you are in a café and having a conversation with a person you love, you will hardly notice other people; and if the color of a wall changes slightly, you are unlikely to observe it. Such blindness in a café cannot be harmful, but when you are on the road, inattentional or change blindness can lead to an accident. In life, your focus (and associated blindness) can define what you can or cannot become and what you perceive in the world. The same world can be perceived in completely different ways, and it depends on your focus.

There is infinite potential in this world, which is usually hidden; however, you can perceive it only if you truly focus on it and take action to bring it into your being. If you do not expect a good change in your life, then the probability of it happening decreases rapidly. Your focus and realistic expectations matter most.

There are endless other optical illusions (distortion or creation of colors, shapes, and meaning as well as other tricks), and the collective evidence of such widespread false impressions of reality that the human brain can weave in an instant suggests that you cannot trust the activity in your head without any objective evidence or practical reason, especially when the stakes are high.

It is hard to draw a fine line between facts and illusions. The conflict between objectivity and subjectivity should be resolved, keeping end goals in mind.

You may or may not encounter optical illusions in daily life, and it does not matter because you benefit from them. However, as soon as you wake up, automatic thoughts and emotions can start pouring into your mind, and each one of them can be subjected to one or more illusions, which can account for a major part of stress or suffering in your life.

Fortunately, other thoughts can bring cognitive illusions to judgment and can stop the associated suffering with them; however, you need something superior than a ruler to detect them and even more powerful cognitive skills to manage them.

The idea that something that is false or unreal but appears to be true or real not only is an interesting fact that surprises you but also is of profound importance, if living life happily and rationally is one of your goals. Visual illusions are related to only one aspect of perception, whereas cognitive illusions are diverse and can infiltrate your every thought.

We will discuss the potential damage, which can be inflicted by the filling-in illusion, in this chapter. Other illusions of thoughts and emotions are discussed throughout the book.

The filling-in illusion of visual perception exposes the many tricks of your brain, and it has a cognitive counterpart too. The tricks of visual perception assist in your survival, but your brain can use the same tricks for your cognitions and emotions, and such use can be equally disturbing for the practical utility of both.

Distortion and creation of information in visual perception is useful because it is not convenient for you to see two black spots whenever you open your eyes.

When your brain uses the filling-in illusion to remember the past or imagine the future, all hell may break loose. To understand why, a brief introduction of the brain and its imperfections is needed; this knowledge is also critical to realize why your brain can turn against you and what you can do about it.

THE HUMAN BRAIN

The human brain is a breathtakingly complex, multitasking, information-processing machine that is woven into the fabric of billions of interconnected neurons and among other know and unknowns, it is ability of your neurons to perceive, process, store, and retrieve information, which seems to give rise to the incredible wonders of the brain.

Neurons are cells, but they are different from the rest of the cells in the human body. A typical neuron has three major parts: the cell body, dendrites, and the axon, as shown in figure 6. The cell body of a neuron contains the genetic material; dendrites receive information from other neurons and transmit it to the cell body; the axon transmits information from the cell body to other neurons, organs, and muscles.

Dendrites look similar to a tree, and the axon is a tail-like structure. The axon is usually protected by an insulating layer of fatty tissue called the myelin sheath, which is similar to the insulation around an electrical wire.

Some neurons differ in their structure to suit the need of a particular location, but the end goal of a neuron is always to handle information.

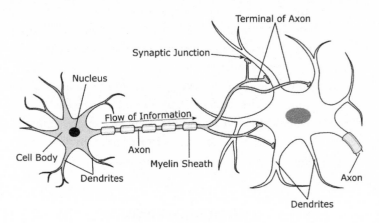

Figure 6
A typical neuron

Neurons do not touch each other, and there is a small synaptic gap between the cell body or dendrites of one neuron and the axon of another neuron. The overall corresponding region or junction is called a synapse. There are about one hundred billion neurons in the human brain, and most neurons have a few thousand synaptic junctions, resulting in a few hundred trillion synapses.

Neurons in the brain need oxygen and nutrients, just like the other cells in the human body, but they also rely on neurotransmitters to transfer information chemically between any two neurons through a synaptic gap. Information inside a neuron, from dendrites to the end of the axon, is transferred by an electrical signal that is protected by the myelin sheath.

Some neurotransmitters and their major areas of influence include the following:

- Dopamine—motivation, emotion, pleasure, motor

- Serotonin—mood, well-being, social dominance, sleep, sex, eating, memory
- Endorphins—reduction in the perception of pain
- GABA (gamma-aminobutyric acid)—mood, anxiety, inhibition
- Norepinephrine—awareness of dangers, vigilance, stress response
- Acetylcholine (ACh)—motor, memory, learning
- Glutamate—excitatory, memory, learning

You need biologically healthy neurons and a delicate balance of neurotransmitters for a healthy brain. A deformity in any biological neural structure or an imbalance of neurotransmitters can change how you perceive, think, feel, and act. Most of the drugs that change your mood manipulate the working mechanism of neurotransmitters.

Agonists are drugs that increase the function of a neurotransmitter, and antagonists are drugs that decrease it. However, drugs unnaturally alter the delicate equilibrium of neurotransmitters, and they have side effects. Natural ways to deal with the problem of fleeting happiness are discussed in detail later. A psychiatrist or psychologist must address any natural imbalance of neurotransmitters.

There are three main types of neurons: sensory neurons, motor neurons, and interneurons. Sensory neurons receive relevant information from the external world through the senses and transfer it to the brain for processing. Motor neurons carry signals from the brain to the muscles to produce movement. Interneurons connect sensory neurons, motor neurons, and other interneurons.

Your spine can also perceive the world and produce movement without your brain's intervention.

Computational power, consciousness, focus, short-term memory, and long-term memory are the fundamental neural resources, and nature has imposed a limit on all of them. The limits of neural resources and their consequences are a recurrent theme of this book and are discussed throughout.

The nervous system is the complete network of neurons in your brain and body, and it can be divided into several physical subsystems. Numerous related neurons and neurotransmitters can work together as a system, and each system can manage a specific task, such as vision, fear, panic, pain, pleasure, and so on. Every system receives or exchanges information with the senses, memory, or other systems or neural structures.

At a higher level, the brain can be logically divided into two systems: fast subconscious and slow conscious. This logical division is discussed later.

You may be wondering why you need to know about the physical or logical structure of the brain. Here is one reason: your brain acts as a whole, but it is actually a set of neural circuits that can act in an inaccurate or incoherent manner, as you have seen in the visual illusions, where one circuit creates an illusion and the other can tell you that it is an illusion. In a similar fashion, some survival circuits in your brain can covert the usual matters of life (or even opportunities) into a matter of life and death; fortunately, other circuits can prevent or manage such absurdity if they are active and strong enough.

There are several other primordial neural circuits in your brain that can be turned on erroneously by your brain, and more on this is discussed later.

What you learn from your experiences becomes a circuit in your brain that can also be triggered in an arbitrary manner. For example, you can acquire bad habits (drug abuse, for example) from your habitat, but your brain may or may not discriminate between good and bad when it decides the activation of addictive self-destructive circuits in an arbitrary manner.

Your brain can also recruit conflicting circuits at the same time, and more on the incoherent absurd activation is also discussed later.

In general, you have several primal as well as learned circuits, which may or may not be helpful. You need to either literally kill the old circuits or develop alternative neural circuits that can prevent or override those that cannot be killed or controlled all the time. We will discuss how to do that later, but awareness of several parts of the brain, and knowing how to make a change in circuits, is critical so that you can realize what is going on in your mind and take corrective action if necessary. This ability alleviates the suffering and primes you for success.

Now that we know a few critical reasons, with more to follow shortly in detail, let's continue our discussion of the neural structure of the brain.

Physically, at a higher level, the brain can be divided into three parts: the hindbrain, the midbrain, and the forebrain, as shown in figure 7.

The hindbrain coordinates the incoming and outgoing information from the spinal cord. The hindbrain (figure 8) can be divided into the medulla, which is responsible for respiration, heart rate, and circulation, the reticular formation, which regulates arousal, sleep, and wakefulness, the cerebellum, which executes fine motor skills, and the pons, which is responsible for relaying information from the cerebellum to rest of the brain.

The midbrain (figure 8) is made from tectum, which orients a living organism in its environment, and tegmentum, which is necessary for arousal and movement. The forebrain controls complex cognitive, perception, emotion, and motor functions. This highest level of the brain can be divided into the subcortical structures and the cerebral cortex. The subcortical structures (figure 9) include the thalamus, hypothalamus, hippocampus, amygdala, and pituitary gland, among others.

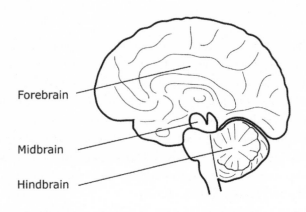

Figure 7
High-level physical structures of the brain

The cerebral cortex is the outermost and most complex layer of the brain, and it is divided into two hemispheres that are connected by the corpus callosum.

The thalamus intercepts and filters the information coming from the senses (except smell) and transfers it to the cerebral cortex. The hypothalamus takes care of hunger, thirst, thermoregulation, and sexual behavior. The hippocampus helps in permanent storage of information from short-term memory to long-term memory. The amygdala is the emotional center of the brain and attaches emotional significance to raw information. The pituitary gland makes different hormones and is the center of the body's hormone system.

The cerebral cortex (figure 10) can be divided into the occipital lobe, which is accountable for visual information processing, the parietal lobe, which oversees perception and makes sense of the world, the temporal lobe, which is critical for memory, understanding, hearing, and language, and the frontal lobe.

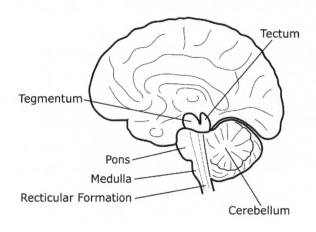

Figure 8
The hindbrain and midbrain

The frontal lobe is responsible for abstract thinking, planning, problem-solving, personality, judgment, self-control, movement, and other higher order functions. The subcortical structures interact with the cerebral cortex through the limbic system, which is the collection of the hypothalamus, the hippocampus, and the amygdala. Overall, there can be several ways to divide the brain into logical or physical systems, but different systems cannot work in isolation. All neural circuits are part of one whole nervous system.

Billions of neurons and trillions of synaptic junctions bring together the information-processing neural circuits into being, and these circuits are responsible for your motivation, perception, cognition, emotion, and action. What the nervous system does is unbelievable, but its creation is far from perfect. Some critical categories of imperfection are introduced next, and each type of imperfection can lead to some kind of illusion. More on each is discussed throughout the book.

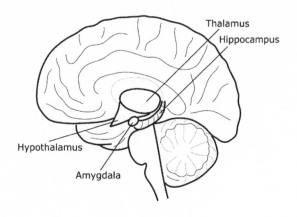

Figure 9
The subcortical structures

IMPERFECTIONS OF THE HUMAN BRAIN

Filters of Meaning

Visual perception is a sensation in the eyes that not only detects lines, curves, and various colors in the environment but also creates automatic, fast, and meaningful mental representation by organizing, recognizing, and interpreting those sensations.

However, this process trades accuracy for speed and meaning for objectivity and thus can produce occasional errors in the otherwise efficient information processing.

The one 3-D image that you see is created by your brain in real time from two upside-down and partially overlapping 2-D images, formed in both of your eyes, with blind spots in each of them. This instant conversion from two different 2-D images to one 3-D image is not exactly the way the outside world is, but it is designed to make sense of the incoming visual information.

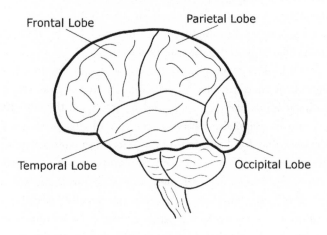

Figure 10
The cerebral cortex

The goal of your vision is to find food, a partner, and predators in the wild; it does not involve seeing an infinitely small electron or a massive galaxy that is millions of light years away. The visual reality that you see is not the accurate or complete objective reality as it is but the way your brain wants you to see it, with survival as the primary motivation. For example, when you see a fruit, you do not see it in its full complexity at the cellular, molecular, atomic, or subatomic level. You see an object that you can eat.

We even give it a short name to further reduce its stunning subatomic complexity, and billions of particles just become an apple. Naming is important because we live in a social world, and names can be used by everyone in a society to recognize the same object or idea.

Similarly, when you see a stick, you see it as a tool with which to pluck a high-hanging fruit or to fight off a predator. All the available information in a fruit or a stick is infinite for your brain, and meaning is what matters most, not the infinite objective facts.

Your brain can function without all the facts (ignoring most of the irrelevant facts is exactly how the brain and its intelligence works) but not without a meaningful motivation, and you are always free to use the facts of science as a survival tool.

Visual illusions could be considered as design features, not as design flaws, because our brains cannot perceive and interpret infinite objective reality, quickly and accurately, at the same time. The brain is designed for survival, and the mental processes that are responsible for lightning-quick perception and meaningful internal representation of the external world assist in our survival.

Perception must be extremely fast and automatic for any practical use, and absolute accuracy is not possible with limited neural resources. Our brains are still extremely efficient in creating perception and assigning meaning to the objects in the external world, but they cannot make the perception perfect and the meaning foolproof.

Meaning and illusion hence cannot be avoided.

The meaning of objects, and of the world itself, is inevitable for survival, and a subjective meaning of your life is needed for you to flourish as well. Meaning is a practical strategy that may or may not be accurate, and a subjective sense of meaning cannot be replaced with a set of objective facts. What you see is infinitely limited and that, too, is manipulated by your brain for meaning. Meaning has its illusions, but it also makes life possible.

Filters of meaning by which your brain discards the irrelevant information give rise to the fundamental focusing illusion.

In general, you perceive things that you pursue, and the rest of the infinite is ignored. Discarding information is useful when it does not matter, but when a complex problem emerges from the underlying unknown, the solution may also lie in the unknown, along with brand-new opportunities.

A Bounded Brain
Out of infinite information available in the universe, sensory

neurons receive only limited information, which is related to your survival. Your eyes can perceive only a tiny part of the vast electromagnetic spectrum, which is enough to find food, shelter, a partner, and predators in the wild.

You cannot see X-rays, UV light, or the rest of the electromagnetic spectrum. You cannot smell every scent and you cannot hear all frequencies. The resolution at which you perceive is also extremely limited.

Neural hardware makes information processing possible, and it provides a platform for cognitive processes to exist, but the neural resources (focus, memory, and computing power) that perceive, encode, store, and retrieve information are bounded.

Neurons working together become neural resources, but there are limited numbers of neurons in your brain, and the computation capability of each neuron is also limited. Your brain's limitations cannot be avoided.

A bounded brain leads to the inevitability of ignorance, and an abnormal anomaly can easily expose the ignorance of hidden information.

You seem to perceive information related to your survival, and you can never be aware of all the infinite unknown, whether your brain has evolved for it or not. You may understand that you do not know all about quantum mechanics, but you can never know what is not known to the collective humanity yet. You can use your imagination to create things in your head, but the history of evolution and the limit of your brain can infiltrate everything that you can imagine.

A subjective sense of reality seems to emerge from biological evolution, and we do not know yet what is beyond our collective objective knowledge of reality.

Absolute accuracy is neither possible with a bounded brain nor always needed for survival and success. All questions cannot be answered, and a delicate balance of objective and subjective reality, which makes your life easier and that of your family and community, is the practical way to define reality.

Some of our thoughts or ideas can make our survival easier, even when they are not verifiable, and some ideas can make our life miserable, even when they seem to be objectively accurate and accuracy or utility of thoughts is not always obvious. Utility matters with meaning when absolute accuracy is not possible.

Even though limited, you can still receive too much information in each moment, and your brain constantly discards most of it. Your finite focus determines what you perceive and you are blind to the rest. As a consequence of a bounded brain, not only can your thoughts or opinions be illusory but also your perception itself is incomplete and biased; and what may look like a disadvantage is actually the source of all hope.

We know almost nothing about the internal and external worlds, and the subliminal strengths of the brain are beyond assumption. There is infinite potential in the external world, and if you decide on a finite long-term purpose in the infinite cosmos and make a plan, your motivation framework can chase it. Only time will tell what you can do.

Sharing of Neural Resources

Although the limited neural faculty puts a limit on the accuracy of your thoughts, and illusory thoughts (or emotions) are often the source of suffering, the sharing of finite cognitive resources, such as focus and short-term memory, among many competing cognitive processes, can further amplify the inaccuracy or utility.

In general, out of many cognitive processes (thoughts in general), only one thought can occupy your consciousness at a time, and if one greedy or compulsive thought (or desire, emotion, and so on) is not freeing up your mind, other critical processes cannot run.

Not all desires can be fulfilled by wishful thinking alone, and if your mind is inhabited by neurotic desires or by the emotional pain caused by unfulfilled desires most of the time, difficult end goals that you desire are least likely to be attained.

When a desire, which is actually useless in itself, does not leave your mind, your problem-solving ability may be useless. In general, you can get what you want (within the bounds of possibility), but if you cannot cognitively detach yourself from your wants, the probability of your success decreases as the complexity of what you want increases.

You usually feel helpless and experience pain when you are possessed by your desires alone, but most of that can be an illusion. Obsessions or compulsions are not happiness.

Evolution of the Brain

The accuracy or usefulness of your cognitions and emotions is also affected by the way the brain has evolved over millions of years.

Your nervous system was not designed at once, but it seems to have evolved from a single cell in the wild. During the evolution of the nervous system, either existing neural structures get bigger or new neural structures are added on top of the existing ones. Primitive structures like the hindbrain and midbrain came first, the cortex came last, and the neural circuits (and people) that were fit for survival remained; the rest disappeared.

The brain has not evolved in the last two million years, and this is one of the most important facts to know in the modern world. Your brain is outdated for the modern wilderness of concrete and information, and it is not easy to be happy or successful in the modern world using the same brain that our ancestors used nearly two million years ago.

In the wild, survival, reproduction, and exploring the unknown, if necessary for both, are the primary goals of life, and the brain is quite sufficient for those tasks. The modern world has lowered our suffering of death and diseases with the help of science and technology, but at the same time, suffering seems to have increased because of the imagination and its interaction with the difficult-to-interpret information.

Animals also have a similar hindbrain and midbrain, but their cortex is very small compared to humans; this cortex is what separates humans from the rest of the animals. The ability to imagine the future and to simulate human emotions primarily comes from the cortex, and, as discussed later, this imagination can be the main source of illusory suffering in modern living.

Your brain does an incredible job of making sense of infinite information with extremely limited neural resources, and it has some innate instincts, along with an amazing ability to learn. These features are likely to be accurate or adaptable under usual circumstances (but not always) and sufficient for survival, generally speaking.

You have several primal circuits that were developed for the wild, but those circuits cannot be made to disappear, even if you do not need them today. Your novel cortex is amazing and problematic at the same time. The circuits that are developed during learning, as you are exposed to your environment, may or may not be for your benefit.

The nervous system runs on several primitive, novel, and learned neural circuits at the same time; however, it is far from perfect when it collaborates with a collection of circuits, each of which is designed to handle a specific task.

Just like the brain creates an illusion of information when it cannot handle it, the brain can activate primitive or irrelevant circuits on occasion for which it has not evolved to or been made for. For example, the stress response (also called the fight-or-flight response), which was meant to deal with predators in the wild, is often activated in the modern world without any predatory threat. Also, as you deal with the complex and ambiguous problems of the modern world, your brain can generate negative and positive cognitions and emotions at the same time by activating different circuits simultaneously.

Ambivalent states of mind do not help and can make matters worse. For example, the unknown is both dangerous and full of potential, and your brain can activate both fear and exploratory circuits, as often happens, for example, when you lose your romantic partner or your job. You can always find a new or better job or partner, but in the moment, it may feel like a matter of life and death. Additional examples are discussed later in the book.

Primitive survival circuits came before the novel cortical circuits in our evolution; in general, these ancient primitive circuits are much more powerful than the circuits of the cortex. Primary circuits run all the basic functions of life and keep you alive. You suffer if they are not happy with the way things are, and you cannot use your cortex effectively. In general, it is only when the survival circuits are satiated that you can think with clarity and be happy.

You have some cortical control over your survival circuits, and to be effective, you need to learn not to panic until there is a real threat to life. Generally speaking, this is one of the most effective ways to be happy in life.

Primitive circuits have the final say, if ambiguity is not resolved by your intellectual cortical circuits soon enough. Survival circuits are not designed for happiness or rationality, and your cortical circuits are usually too lazy or not developed enough to deal with the subcortical structures.

Along with the objective behavior of the nervous system (the stress response, for example), you can also learn subjective behavior from your environment. Your brain can also activate a learned behavior in an unreliable manner. Your brain can learn complex things, and it can also learn computational shortcuts (rules of thumb) on the basis of cues. Sometimes emotions are also neural shortcuts when a perfect solution cannot be computed.

Several examples of the pitfalls of innate and learned circuits are introduced later in the book, and we will see how activation of irrelevant circuits can make you suffer.

You must come up with your own cognitive shortcuts, which can be applied to most cases, to manage the automated motivation, cognition, emotion, and action of your brain. A few such cognitive shortcuts are discussed later, along with the importance of detachment (cognitive defusion) from your cognitions and emotions.

Overall, the content of your consciousness can be activated in a highly unreliably manner because of the evolution of the brain, and such illusory activation can be miserable without any authentic reason.

Physically Wired Circuits

Neural circuits are wired physically in your brain. A learned element of the motivation framework (perception, motivation, action, cognition, imagination, and emotion) is an efficient wiring of associated neural circuits with it, and such efficient neural wiring usually takes time. Unwanted learning may always stay with you because it is not easy to physically remove its neural wiring. Learning new things, which can override or control the unwanted counterpart, takes time. Some behaviors can be learned in an instant, but they are rare.

Overall, learning or unlearning is not easy, and learned things can make you suffer until they are controlled or overridden by the newly developed circuits. Killing old circuits and developing new ones are usually painful, and that is why change is difficult.

So far, we have outlined the primary categories of imperfections of the brain, and each type of imperfection can lead to several cognitive illusions and challenges. The categories of cognitive illusions are defined next, and examples of each are introduced throughout the book.

COGNITIVE ILLUSIONS

In general, illusion is an error in the neural information processing where either subjective experience deviates from the objective reality or the utility of your cognition, action, and emotion does not serve your motivation.

However, our experiences are bounded, and the perceived objective reality is not the absolute actuality—at least not today. Therefore, objectivity may be an illusion as well. This book is focused on illusions, which influence the hedonic motivation and can prevent you from flourishing.

Cognitive illusions are systematic illusions of cognitions or errors of thoughts. Delusions are rigid and false beliefs that are maintained in spite of their logical absurdity. Cognitive fallacy is failing to apply obvious logic, and because of cognitive bias, we draw conclusions or have beliefs where logical evidence is either insufficient or absent.

Usual errors in thinking may arise from wishful thinking, inferior understanding of the world, distorted reasoning, and usual forgetting, and they account for cognitive distortions, which do not apply to all. Cognitive illusion, fallacies, and biases differ from cognitive distortions because they are automatic, systematic, and predictable for most.

For the sake of simplicity, in this book, all kinds of cognitive errors or shortcuts are called illusions, including the flawed emotional feedback of pain and pleasure.

Illusions of visual perception are helpful, but thoughts have even more complex origins than vision, and each of your thoughts is also subjected to illusion. Some of the illusions are not errors but rather tricks of your brain to make your life easier. Some illusions do not matter, but others can cause people to die by suicide or to live a stressed, depressed, anxious, nihilistic, or miserable life.

Cognitive illusions matter because cognitions can direct motivation and other constituents of consciousness. For example, thoughts can even override the fundamental motivation of survival and can cause people to die by suicide, which can be the end result of just one cognitive illusion.

Difficulty in life may be real or illusory, but as long as we are alive and biologically healthy, there is always a realistic hope. Nearly eight hundred thousand people die by suicide every year, and a few million attempt it. Animals do not seem to suffer in such a way, and they are not gifted or cursed with the human brain and its feelings. Emotions in our imagination can be illusory, and knowledge of an ambiguous or deceptive nature of imagination is critical for a thriving life.

There are hundreds of objective and subjective illusions of thoughts and emotions, and introducing them all is beyond the scope of this book. Only the most common ones that affect your health and happiness are discussed here.

Now that we have an overview of brain and its imperfections and illusions, we can come back to the filling-in illusion of cognition and emotion. You will be surprised to see how all hell may break loose because of just one illusion.

THE FILLING-IN ILLUSION

The filling-in illusion exerts influence on the memories of the past, the perception of the present, and the imagination of the future. Such meddling can be downright damaging for your existence.

Memory is a remarkable thing, and even though most of it seems real, it can be illusory. The human brain does not have enough long-term memory to store countless life experiences, and most have too much information associated with them. Your brain stores only a few key details of your experiences in your long-term memory—these are generally the most intense moments and the end of an episode of experiences—and ignores everything else.

When you try to recall the past, the brain fills in the previously ignored information that it did not store with information available in the present. This happens quietly and quickly, without your awareness, and creates an illusion of memory in which you are deluded into a belief that you have recalled your memories exactly as you experienced them firsthand.

Memory recall is dependent on the information available in the present, and because the present is always different from the past (no two moments in the universe can be exactly the same; in fact, you can never be certain about the present either at the quantum level), we sometimes could recall things that we actually did not experience. In other words, information acquired after an experience can change the memory of that experience.

For example, psychological pain of the past can disappear in an instant when something exceptional happens in your life; and when you fall in love or emerge victorious after years of agonizing action, the pain of the past does not matter in the moment, regardless of its intensity. Similarly, if someone you trusted betrays you, all your memories of the past can change with the flick of a switch, as if there was nothing positive.

Your memories, which look like objective facts, can be converted from hell to heaven or from heaven to hell in an instant, as hidden opportunity or ever-present underlying chaos reveals itself.

An underlying assumption—that memories are always stored with complete detail or recalled with absolute accuracy—is just an illusion.

The filling-in trick of your brain also influences your forecasting of the future.

If memory recall is reweaving a little saved information from the past with the abundant available information in the present, then the imagination of the future is mostly projecting current available information onto the future. The imagination of the future not only is predicting what and when something will happen but also is trying to experience your emotions in advance, over a period of time, for different future outcomes.

Imagination is an extremely powerful cognitive feature because it lets you live in a simplified simulation of the objective world, in your head, without trying out your ideas in the real world. However, simulation of your brain is imperfect and is infected by the fundamental focusing illusion.

Supercomputers can predict the future better than the human brain because they have a lot of memory and computing power. However, the prediction ability of supercomputers is also bounded, and they do not have natural intelligence, thoughts, and emotions like humans do, at least not today. Computers can also store a lot of information because of the ever-expanding long-term memory, but it is not infinite, and infinite information cannot be managed by supercomputers.

Your brain does not have enough long-term memory to store all your experiences, and it does not have enough computing power and working memory to imagine the future without vagueness. For example, when you get married, you usually imagine a future with boundless happiness, but sooner or later, your honeymoon ends and reality sets in, telling you that your imagination of the future was an overrated illusion.

Your brain can do many complex things needed for your survival, but it cannot predict the weather or the outcome of any other complex set of systems, and it cannot multiply two big numbers without a paper and pen. The nervous system can also predict pain and pleasure from the past and present, but, as discussed later, most of those hedonic forecasts are focusing illusions, concentrating on only a tiny part of the information and ignoring the infinite.

For the human brain, perception of the present is most accurate, and memory is much clearer than the prediction of the future. The implications of this fact are manifold.

Available information, depending on your mental focus or circumstances, starts a cascading effect, which infiltrates thoughts of the past, present, or future. For example, an entrepreneur struggling to survive the brutal process of entrepreneurship, or a person struggling with depression, divorce, or any other difficulty, could paint the cruel present over their entire future, where hope is beyond the horizon and pain is all that is visible. However, with the knowledge of the filling-in illusion, people can find solace in the fact that with enough mental and physical action, the future can be made different and be brighter than the present.

Hope is almost always real, even when it seems unreal. More examples, along with the realistic strengths of your brain, are discussed later in the book.

Although some people have a neurobiological deficiency of some sort and grapple with various psychological disorders as a result, healthy people can also become depressed or anxious, at least at some point in their lives, because of the brutality of the being.

The filling-in illusion changes the way you think and feel about the past or the future in an illusory way. When life is hard, the filling-in illusion can ensure that you drown in the sea of misery and stay there for a long time, maybe forever.

Your brain can never grasp the infinite information, and the future will reveal itself in absolute detail only when you are in it, not before. Possibilities are open for you always, no matter what has happened in the past, provided that you are capable of the usual mental and physical action. A future without hope is usually an illusion, as long as you are open to life, keep learning, and do not stop.

In reality, you can never know what you can do unless you try again and again. Going after difficult and complex goals, voluntarily, changes how your nervous system works. Such a strategy can activate the challenge response, the dopaminergic system, and your inactive genes to generate new proteins.

When you deal with the uncertain or unknown, as you may often do, your brain tends to project the known onto the unknown and certainty onto uncertainty. When times are extremely tough, memories of the past and the imagination of the future are usually infected by the brutality of the present and the known. When we feel the ultimate pain, the past and future both look bleak, even when there were magnificent things in the past and even when the future can be made spectacular in time.

The filling-in illusion infuses irrationality and insanity into your consciousness, turning temporary setbacks or challenges into a permanent reality. The filling-in and other illusions can trick you into believing that current circumstances are all there is, all there were, and all there will be, but you can learn not to trust your thoughts. Learning to intercept and direct your automatic thoughts and emotions on the basis of their accuracy or utility is a fundamental cognitive skill you can develop to live a life that does not betray itself.

OVERCONFIDENCE

General intelligence is the ability to solve the complex problems of life. Animals can solve simple problems of survival as well. Neural efficiency (above-average short-term memory, high nerve conduction velocity, low reaction time, and other neural factors) leads to higher levels of intelligence.

If you have a healthy nervous system, it is interesting to know what illusions can do to your intelligence. The IQ test is a popular method to measure general intelligence, and such tests include images. However, if you design a test in such a way that most of the images include a visual illusion of some sort, the score could be close to zero.

When we think about intelligence, we usually think of it as being accurate or creative, but human intelligence is not about accuracy all the time, and creativity is coming up with several ideas so that at least one can work. Natural human intelligence is also an ability to come to a speedy conclusion for a motivation, and creative imagination of the human brain can be used for self-destruction without a genuine motivation.

Perception is a part of human intelligence, and artificial intelligence has yet to achieve this feat as we do, because in the objective world, there is no moral hierarchy without a motivation, and the available information is infinite. Without a motivation, a machine cannot decide what to focus on in the infinite, and a motivation is a subjective affair.

Ignorance is inevitable for intelligence to exist alongside a motivation framework and a bounded brain. Because your brain does not inform you when it deludes you, overconfidence is also inevitable.

A planning fallacy is an excellent example of overconfidence in different domains at the same time. Experts, who think that they have the knowledge and skills to predict and validate the timeline and resources needed to finish a complex project, are almost always wrong. In general, experts usually underestimate the time and effort needed for the completion of a complex project by a great degree; you hear about this in the news all the time. A public infrastructure project is usually delayed again and again, with additional costs. Even after completion, many of them fail to achieve the planned purpose of the project. Overconfidence may not be apparent in simple things, but the complexity or an anomaly can expose it vividly.

Overconfidence is a positive illusion and it often works, but it can backfire when things get tough. A naive, overblown sense of self-importance can work if you have perfect genes and a perfect environment, but life is unfair, and underlying chaos can pop up at any time, without warning. Naivety is not going to help when you deal with multiple complex problems at the same time, and overconfidence will then have a profound negative effect on your well-being.

Interestingly, hopelessness may seem like a lack of confidence, but as far as there is no serious biological disability, it can be overconfidence in the delusional thoughts and emotions. However, it is not easy to control thoughts and emotions, even with the awareness of their faults (what can be done about it is discussed later).

Ignorance and arrogance are integral features of your brain, and awareness of this fact matters the most if minimizing pain in your life is one of your goals.

Visual illusions reveal that in the process of creating a single 3-D image from two 2-D images, your brain is free to change the meaning or representation of various objects in the vision field. Your vision seems authentic, but it is not as credible as it appears to be. The accuracy of your thoughts about pain or pleasure, from your experiences in the past or from your imagination of the future, is usually incredibly thin.

Illusions are a recurrent theme of this book, because only if you can control the self-inflicted, avoidable suffering of the deceptive or obsessive thoughts and emotions, can you use the stellar strengths of your brain to live a life free from self-deception and one that is full of joy.

Illusions may try to project unhappiness, hopelessness, misery, and defeat over all your life, but you have the right to repudiate such absurdity and to bring realistic hope back into your life with rational and realistic cognitions that can direct or override all other elements of the motivation framework for your welfare, one way or another.

Formal education and the media do not teach you the science of the brain. You prefer not to create doubt in the automatic thoughts and emotions pouring into your consciousness, without realizing that they can be illusory, irrational, or, in extreme cases, can create psychological suffering that does not seem to die.

A thought bringing other thoughts to reason and under control, as a result of knowing that they can be wrong, is the backbone of intellectual rationality, which institutes tranquility in life, as opposed to the unchecked automatic thoughts, which can unleash relentless misery.

Thinking must be put to work to monitor and correct itself.

DUALITY, EQUANIMITY, AND COURAGE

Hedonic motivation seems simple and straightforward: just pursue pleasure and prevent pain, and you are done. Feel pleasure whenever you want to feel it, at least when you consciously want it, and remove pain from your life, at least psychologically. But is it that simple, and can you not feel pain at all but simply pleasure all the time?

Sometimes life is simple and pleasure is all you feel. When everything in your life is going great, you feel good, without any conscious cognitive effort.

But what happens when your life is not so great, or you are going through excruciating psychological or physical pain? There is nothing much you can do with the physical pain, apart from taking medications, but can you turn off your psychological misery anytime you wish and be happy?

You know the answer.

You may seek happiness, but one of the most surprising and brutal facts of life is that your hedonic quest can easily and quietly become an eternal source of pain, not pleasure.

You do not need to refer to any sophisticated scientific study for evidence of the paradoxical nature of hedonic motivation; the evidence is all around you. For ages, people have used and abused people and substances for happiness, and the smartphone has become the new substance.

You can find people on street corners with alcohol in their blood, juggling cigarettes, coffee, and their mobile phones, trying to find happiness. Maybe people can find happiness from drugs and other substances, but such pleasure does not last, and it often leads to more pain in the long run.

We cannot always blame people for such struggle because cognitive fitness is not taught in schools, which can prevent all this. What is needed is not always obvious in the world of infinite information, when people also struggle with the suffering of life.

Conventional wisdom or group thinking, ignoring the widespread evidence, tells you to hoard money (if you can), buy material things, and be happy. It seems simple, but is it?

They do not tell you how much money or how many things are enough for your happiness. Maybe they do not know what they are talking about, or maybe they just want to use you, or maybe it's something else. Whatever the reason, you may believe in such baloney and keep living these monetary delusions, whereas some highly successful people kill themselves by drug overdose, when they end up using drugs for happiness, after endless material things bought by their money are rendered useless.

The importance of money for survival in the modern world is obvious, but money alone cannot guarantee happiness.

Clearly, the realization of your hedonic motivation is not easy, even with money, materialism, power, fame, substance abuse, social security, social media, or any other popular belief, and it can comfortably make you run on a hedonic treadmill, as you frantically search for happiness, with discreet pauses, but your run never ends.

If the pursuit of happiness is not easy, can we at least minimize our suffering with relative ease?

The answer to this question is also paradoxical.

In general, people who can tolerate the inevitable pain feel less overall pain in life, in the long run. People who are too sensitive toward pain often suffer much more than is destined for them. It is also observed that courage to voluntarily face the inevitable suffering of life reduces the intensity of overall pain, and as we will discuss later, courage can also activate positive and powerful parts of your brain.

The hedonic principle cleverly conceals its paradoxical persona, and what we do not realize is that a desire to experience happiness is noble, but a compulsive desire can easily be adverse to happiness itself. The inability to confront and endure pain patiently can intensify every type of psychological pain in your life.

As noted earlier, the purpose of emotional pain and pleasure is to provide feedback on your actions in the real world or in the imagination. Action is necessary for survival and the pursuit of purpose.

There is a reason for the existence of each of the elements in the motivation framework, and there is a reason for the motivation itself. To find a purpose for your life, you need reason, and this reason separates a motivation (for your existence) from a desire.

Desire can arise automatically, without any authentic reason; however, a purpose for your life is a well-thought-out motivation and has subjective reasons. Desires are usually arbitrary and have pleasure as the end goal, whereas a motivation is defined with reason, and the end goal is survival and the pursuit of purpose.

Surprisingly, you experience authentic happiness when you do not beg for it and when you pursue a purpose other than happiness itself.

Desires, which pursue pleasure instead of purpose, ironically result in much more pain than pleasure and pursuit of a purpose can let you experience authentic happiness, without even asking for it. The ability to endure pain (negative emotional feedback) patiently and to detach yourself from negative emotions is one of the best ways to alleviate pain and to use the pain to your advantage.

Why the contents of your consciousness can be arbitrary (including your desires for pleasure) and why a purpose in life is the best way to deal with hedonic motivation is discussed later. In this chapter, the psychology of pain and pleasure is introduced, which explains why the problem posed by your hedonic motivation is paradoxical in nature and what you can do about it.

THE DESIRE FOR PLEASURE

The desire to experience pleasure is the underlying behavior that governs us all to facilitate our survival, using reward as its currency. Despite the fundamental importance of desires, they can lead to a person's decline. This suggestion seems unusual at first, but the fact that nearly 40 percent of premature deaths in the United States are partially attributed to desire regulation tells us that decline caused by desires could result in our early demise.

Uncontrollable desires can not only cut short our existence but also are toxic for our intellectual cognitive capabilities.

The psychology of desire, which is introduced in this section, sheds some light on the life cycle of desire and explains how, despite their innocent intent, desires can add to and amplify the troubles in our life.

Desires may delude you by asserting that they can make your life happy forever, but in reality, that is rarely true. Desires alone are not enough, and sometime months of painstaking work is required before the probability of your success turns into possibility.

If your wishes are granted (which does not happen often), you experience actual happiness from the consumption of a reward, but sooner or later, that happiness fades away. Fulfilled desires tend to lose their appeal with time, and as it becomes increasingly difficult to gain pleasure from the same reward, you long for another desire, with the obvious hope of finding enduring happiness once again. When the onset of that brand-new happiness ends, the viscous cycle of desire begins again.

Desire (wanting) may lead to happiness (liking) from the consumption of the reward (if you get what you want), but acquired happiness from that recent reward decreases over time, until it completely disappears or becomes normal (habituation, adaptation and satiation). This dwindling happiness compels you to create and chase a new desire, initiating a cycle that never seems to end.

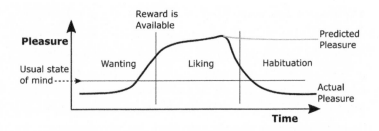

Figure 11
The life cycle of pleasure (for a fulfilled desire) over time

Figure 11 represents a life cycle of pleasure that can be experienced from a fulfilled desire. The interesting thing in the graph of experienced pleasure from a reward over time is the inaccuracy in the emotional prediction. Your imagination usually tells you that pleasure will last forever, with the same intensity, once you get the reward, but this prediction is often an illusion. With time, habituation or other neural circuits kill your pleasure, and you go back to your usual state of mind. If your desire is not fulfilled, you can easily live in the emotional pain of imagined and illusory permanent happiness.

Liking is the only thing that is generally good about a desire, as long as what you want is not self-destructive but authentic. Illusions of wanting, a dearth of liking, and the brutality of habituation are discussed next.

WANTING: THINKING ABOUT REWARDS

Desire is wanting—in other words, thinking about pleasure but not experiencing the actual pleasure.

Neuroscience suggests that wanting is motivation to approach the reward, think about the reward, or be reminded of the reward by internal or external cues, whereas liking is the actual pleasurable experience or hedonic effect of the reward. Both are different neurobiological mechanisms because they are registered in different areas of the brain by different mental processes.

Desire is hedonic forecasting in time; liking is enjoying what you already have, without any wanting. Desire is wanting, not liking, and this fact makes all the difference.

You have a desire for a better future, and this is a noble and necessary goal, but when desire makes you restless and unhappy in the present, diminishing your chances of liking the past, present, or future, all hell may break loose. Providing a fully comprehensive and detailed description of the imperfections of thinking associated with wanting is beyond the scope of this book, but a brief introduction follows that describes how your nervous system becomes frenzied when it runs on desires.

Cognitive Illusions Associated with Desires

You possess a highly sophisticated experience simulator, which is a recent gift to you from Mother Nature, and you use it for hedonic forecasting—predicting future pain or pleasure from past experiences. You first try to predict how the future will unfold and then, using your neural simulator, you try to forecast the type and intensity of your emotions associated with your predictions, over time.

The ability to conceptualize the future, predict it, and simulate the emotional experiences is a revolutionary ability of the human brain, which lets you plan, sacrifice the present, and work hard for a better future. However, given the brain's limits, it cannot predict the future flawlessly. You can rationalize this fact easily, but it is the hedonic prediction that may appear authentic, even when it is deeply flawed.

Your brain does a terrific job of simulating some experiences perfectly, but it can also do a poor job of simulating other emotions erratically over time and an even poorer job when it fails to tell you that several of its hedonic predictions are full of errors. Some of the errors, limitations, and cognitive processes that make it harder for your simulator to work accurately are discussed next.

Impact Bias

You predict the type of emotion felt from a distant event more or less accurately, but it is the intensity and duration of that feeling, over time, that is usually inaccurately predicted. The overall effect of emotional events is often overrated, and such exaggeration can have grave consequences.

You may predict boundless happiness from your marriage to the love of your life, and you are partially correct. Initial happiness after a marriage is usually warranted, but the mistaken part of your prediction is the assumed permanence of your initial emotions. The intensity of your initial feelings usually fades with time.

Even the most important things in life can be converted into nothing as time progresses. The things that once gave you happiness are highly unlikely to give you continual happiness, and the sameness sets in.

Sometimes you may live with the errors of your predictions, but these errors become a psychological burden when you amplify predicted happiness from a future event so out of proportion that your overrated forecast turns into a miserable obsession. Obsessions are usually not comfortable; they not only make you suffer but also undermine your problem-solving cognitive ability.

You may have lived in peace in a small village a thousand years ago (assuming you did not have any chronic disease and had family, food, and security), but today your peace may be robbed by the exaggerations of pleasure from endless materialistic things or from some other possibility of the modern world.

You also degrade your health by the stress and misery that come into your life when you obsessively want the overrated happiness of a luxury but cannot attain it. Pursuit of a better future is a good goal, and a must in most cases, but not at the expense of your health and not because of an illusory dramatization of reality.

You can also extrapolate erroneous exaggerations of pain or pleasure backward in time and create pain in the present anytime you wish; negative exaggerations are even worse. We will later discuss why your brain is biased toward negativity.

Overrated thoughts of pain or pleasure over time can make you miserable in the present or maybe even forever. An obsession with happiness is not happiness, and overrated obsessions can ensure that you never get the thing you are obsessed about. More on the negative effect of obsessions on your cognitive performance is discussed later.

Hot/Cold Empathy Gaps

You experience empathy gaps when you try to predict your emotional reaction to a distant emotional or motivational state, which is different from the psychological state at the time of prediction.

Cold to hot empathy gaps can cause you to overrate current cold states (such as depression, stress, boredom, and anxiety), and as a result, you can pessimistically predict the probable future hot states (such as love, joy, pride, peace, and happiness). Hot to cold empathy gaps make you forget that the current hot emotional or motivational state is temporary. For example, when you fall in love, you almost cannot imagine a future without the magical warmth of romantic love, and when you are depressed, it is almost impossible to imagine a future full of happiness.

When trying to predict the future, a person in a depressed state is unlikely to imagine a blissful one. Because a beautiful future may be unthinkable, the person may not even try to solve the problem, but without any corrective action, depression can go on. Knowing that a future without hope is usually an illusion and that with effort one can feel good again, even though it is unimaginable in the present, can prevent such misery.

It may be painful to keep working when there seems to be no hope, but this pain slowly moves you upward and is far better than the pain of sitting in a sea of illusions and doing nothing. The inevitability and utility of pain is presented later in this chapter.

Life is generally not that bad for everyone but only if delusions can be diluted. Not giving up is almost always a superior strategy than giving up. Even a tiny improvement every day is usually enough for things to get much better in a few months or years.

A setback or euphoria is almost always temporary, and assuming permanent defeat or taking a substantial risk is not a great strategy. Your brain will habituate your euphoria, and some setbacks can be magnified into illusory permanence.

Empathy gaps can produce significant errors in decision-making when you imagine pain and pleasure from emotions that you currently do not have. Relying on your emotionally charged state, hot or cold, when you make a significant decision for your life can cost you in the present and in the future.

Immune Neglect

We tend to overestimate the emotional effect of negative events. For example, in the case of a breakup, you can unconsciously focus on the flaws of your ex-partner and feel better sooner than you predict.

Your brain has a powerful cognitive immune system, made up of various cognitive processes that help to reduce the effect of suffering inflicted by life. These sense-making processes, such as self-affirmation, self-deception, positive illusions, motivated reasoning, dissonance reduction, and defense mechanisms, among others, cannot erase pain from your life, but life would be much more painful without them.

Despite its inclination toward negativity, your brain does provide a buffer against major setbacks. However, when many things go wrong in your life at the same time, then you can be in real trouble because your psychological immune system struggles to prevent a dooming depression and other mental disorders.

Ordinization Neglect
Because of the sense-making processes, the positive effect of novel events can also disappear sooner than you predict. For example, a promotion may not be exciting for long because the sense-making process will advise you that you deserved it. On the other hand, you may keep waiting for a promotion obsessively, deluding yourself with the prolonged pleasure of promotion.

Misconstrual Problem
Sometimes we can predict the wrong event. For example, a woman might imagine the birth of her first child as a trouble-free delivery, followed by a wonderful bonding time with the baby, but in reality, it could be very different—the birth painful and the child demanding for years.

Duration Neglect
The peak of pain or pleasure matters most, along with the end; the overall duration is often neglected. For example, you may assume that all your memories of happiness from future experiences are going to be saved, but your brain has limited long-term memory, and it stores only key details (the peaks and the end, in general)

and ignores the rest.

Focusing Illusion

This is the mother of all illusions and it infects everything, including your wanting.

Your prediction of the future, or hedonic forecasting, can never be accurate always because of your ability to focus on only a tiny part of the information available and being blind to everything else. No matter how hard you try, you may come closer, but you can never forecast all the possible entangled outcomes of your wanting. Reality reveals itself vividly when you are in it—not before and not in your forecasts.

When you think about pain and pleasure in the future, or in the past, your brain creates an extremely limited subjective world in your head, and as you focus on a few things responsible for pain or pleasure, other unimaginable infinite things are ignored, but they will influence your future positive and negative emotions.

It was outlined earlier that your neural resources (focus, memory, and computing power to process information) are limited; therefore, out of the infinite information available in the universe, what you perceive is restricted, and your focus can direct your consciousness to hold the finite data; the rest is ignored at that time.

You can never think about everything at a given time. You may be partially or fully objective about one thing at a time, but there are several systems that govern the brain and the world. These systems do not work in isolation all the time.

The interplay of various internal and external systems (known and unknown) is extremely complicated, and high-resolution, multidimensional critical thinking is exceptionally difficult. Your focus simplifies the complexity by concentrating on one thing and ignoring everything else, but it also introduces a fundamental focusing illusion into your thinking.

We need strategies or heuristics (well-designed cognitive

shortcuts or rules of thumb) that are likely to be true in most cases for the extremely complicated and intermingled matters of life. As far as your hedonic motivation is concerned, if you have good health, family and friends, and socioeconomic security, your life is already good.

The cognitive illusions of wanting, with a focusing illusion being in the forefront, may suggest otherwise, but in most cases, it is a lie. You can short-circuit all the disheartening cognitive illusions with this simple fact of life.

There are several other illusions associated with wanting, but providing a full list is beyond the scope of this book. Thinking about the pleasure that could be experienced from brand-new things in the future is fine, but problems arise when your thinking becomes distorted or obsessive.

Illusions of wanting can make your life difficult and miserable, especially if what you want is going to take months to materialize. Critical thinking is required, with cognitive clarity, in such cases.

It is extremely hard to say what can cause lasting pain or pleasure, but as long as you have health and human connection, nothing else matters as much as you think. Predicting pain and pleasure is never as simple as it seems.

Errors in predicting the future, which are part of desire or wanting, may lead to errors in decision-making. As desires become more and more intense, cognitive errors become more biased and distorted, leading to even more errors, confusion, and suffering.

As a result, when the going gets tough, your brain can ensure that your life becomes worse. Unrelenting physical pain paves the way for real suffering, but most of the prolonged psychological pain can be purely illusory, which is the recurring theme of this book.

An awareness of flawed hedonic forecasting is the first step in erasing most of the avoidable emotional pain in life related to desires. It is critical to assimilate and grasp the fact that what you see or think can be misguided and untrue and can appear as undeniable and genuine in existence.

When you realize that your desires can be illusory, you strip their supreme power over you. It becomes easier to control them, which otherwise could be perceived as truth. Your brain can also convert your usual desires into a matter of life and death.

Cognitive illusions of desires give a false impression of reality—they are as unreal as illusions of your vision. One desire (or assumption, thought, or belief) that is not in line with the objective reality of the internal and external worlds is enough to wipe out any probability of peace or hope in your life.

Care should be exercised when you trust your desires blindly.

The Negative Effect of Desires on Your Cognitive Performance

The second significant problem with desires is that they can have a negative effect on your cognitive performance. This is because uncontrollable desires can compete with other concurrent cognitive tasks for such limited and shared cognitive resources as working memory and attention.

For most people, life is not a fairy tale, and we struggle to find a comforting place between order and chaos.

Advanced cognitive skills (for example, learning from failures, the ability to endure pain, creativity, critical thinking, abstract reasoning, decision-making) can always help you to find solutions. However, as desires grow in intensity or number, they continue to occupy critical cognitive resources, in turn leaving less (or may be no) room for the execution of actual problem-solving cognitive processes.

A desire in itself may not be enough, and advanced knowledge and cognitive skills may be required to get what you desire. However, in the worst case, desires can completely hijack your ability to reason and think clearly; paradoxically, a desire can become an enemy of itself.

Desires lessen cognitive scope and narrow attention, which are required to find a broad range of solutions. Desires lead to tunnel vision and crowd out other self-regulatory behaviors and reflective thoughts. Because a happy brain is more efficient than an unhappy or stressed brain, unpleasant states of mind arising from unfulfilled desires further degrade your cognitive efficiency.

When instant gratification is not possible, solutions are not obvious and critical thinking is required. Wishful thinking or out-of-control desires can make the situation worse. Overall, desires can make you intellectually inefficient, pushing the very thing that you desire away from you, when the thing that you want is not easy to get.

Desires Can Make You Blind

We have discussed how your focus can make you blind visually because of the limited cones in your tiny fovea. Similarly, desires can ensure that you are blind to all other positive and powerful cognitive processes or information, if your focus is completely consumed by wanting and wishful thinking.

Desires Can Invite Behavioral Problems

Desires can lead to addiction, temptation, impulsive or aggressive behavior, want-should conflict, ambivalence, and cognitive dissonance. Although some of these states are a great source of misery, not only for those who are suffering but also for those who are close to them, other such states can be bring discomforts in life and start a struggle between wanting and self-control.

People may even use biased motivated reasoning and heuristics to license self-control failures that are caused by these uncomfortable states—for example, allowing yourself to smoke, drink, or overeat because you are feeling bad.

The desire to self-disclose is one reason for today's social media addiction that could add more unhappiness to life for those who do not engage in face-to-face social interactions.

Anger may arise when you do not get what you want, but anger narrows attention and facilitates aggressive behavior, which generally is not helpful for anyone. In the worst case, aggression can ruin your life very easily.

Many can suffer from neurobiological conditions, but a never-ending desire for happiness can easily be the cause of substance abuse and obesity (and other similar mental and physical conditions) in otherwise fit people.

The desire to feel good at any time can be fulfilled instantly in certain cases, when desired objects are easily available, such as food and cigarettes, but it can also give rise to various health problems associated with obesity and cancer. Having a desire to be happy all the time (or having an assumption that something can lead to permanent happiness) is not happiness and cannot lead to happiness by itself; such desire can instead lead to continual pain.

Controlling Wanting

Wanting does not always lead to liking. It may be experienced better or worse than the actual experience itself, and it depends on the countless cues in the internal and external worlds. For example, smokers may find that thinking about smoking is more pleasurable than smoking itself. This is true for other addictions or desires as well.

Flight crews may experience more cravings for smoking near airports than while they are in flight, and men may approach anything rewarding after looking at pictures of bikini-clad models. Electrode stimulation of wanting regions of the brain does not necessarily give rise to pleasant states and could also induce anxiety or even paranoia.

What you want in any moment is not always your conscious choice, and it is manipulated by your brain from internal and external cues. Thoughts and emotions can arise automatically from environmental cues, and you need self-awareness to monitor them and self-control to manage them. The importance of self-control is discussed in the next chapter.

Crazy Cravings

Cravings can be crazy. When you crave something, your imagination activates your memory by adding known and unknown, real and imaginary, flavors to your experience of craving. Because you do not have what you want in the moment, you cannot help but use your imagination and memory to create virtual moments in your head, where you and your craving meet each other. Pain seems to disappear and pleasure is all that lasts when you encounter your cravings in your mind. You automatically assume that this is how it will be in reality, if only somehow you can attain it.

The movie created by your memory and imagination plays in your head again and again, making your cravings even stronger and more realistic. When time and the complexities of the world stand between your cravings and yourself, the cravings start to become compulsive and tend to take your comfort away. This discomfort may last for days and years until reality eases on you, if it ever does, giving you what you craved for so long and restoring comforts to your life again.

This is when the craziness of cravings becomes apparent.

The script of your memory and imagination that existed in your mind for a long time is tested against the script that life has for you in reality. Sooner or later, you realize that both are different. A thing that you may have desired for years becomes nothing in a matter of months, and you may feel disgusted by the sameness that remains. Your disgust disappears when life strikes again and takes that thing back from you, and you go back to your state of craving.

It is possible that you cannot live comfortably, with or without the same thing.

You Cannot Always Get What You Want

Finally, you cannot always get what you want. To feel the actual pleasure of reward, you first must have what you want. Discrepancies between what you want and what you actually have can cause your emotional downfall.

Desires that are in conflict with the laws of the universe are dead on arrival, and lifelong disappointments are their rewards. For example, people and circumstances in the external world can at no time be directly in your control, and a desire to control everything external can never be fulfilled.

In addition, it is difficult to control your own mind; complete cognitive control over your own neural circuits is not always possible. Similarly, you cannot always experience happiness. Pain is an integral part of life, and it will be there always.

Mother Nature, society, and yourself all have positive and negative elements; the control that you can exercise outside or inside is too limited.

You can influence internal and external worlds within these limits; however, opportunities are also endless in this world. Difficult goals, which are wrapped in complexity, may take years to materialize with no guarantee of success. As your goals become increasingly complicated, you may need to do more work with intellectual cognitive clarity, but out-of-control desires are the enemy of your intellect.

While some work for what they want, others want everything without moving a finger. Some work and can get what they want, and some are betrayed by the self, family, society, and nature. Overall, desires for pleasure know no bounds, not all desires are realistic or authentic, and you cannot always get what you want.

Wanting may not be enough, and what you want is not always easy, constructive, or in your direct control. Wanting is good when it is possible and helpful, but when the going gets tough, untamed desires bring down your cognitive performance and your ability to reason; induce biased and distorted thinking; lead to great discomforts and self-control failures; and may hijack your brain completely, making it harder or impossible for you to get what you want.

LIKING THE REWARD

Liking is the real and authentic pleasure of a reward, as it is available in the present, without any predictions or hedonic simulations of pain or pleasure from the past or future.

Liking is generated in the hedonic hotspots in the brain. These pleasure generators in the brain are not easily available and they are fragile. To create an episode of intense pleasure, a whole network of these hedonic hotspots should be activated together, and even a single inactive hotspot can prevent bliss.

Pleasure is not merely a sensation of sense but something that our brain adds to those experiences. All the pleasure centers of the brain turning on at the same time is an unlikely event. This neuroscientific finding suggests that intense pleasures are relatively rare.

Wanting a reward is the first step that may lead to consumption of a reward, but for the consumption to happen, the reward must be available first. Wanting alone cannot give you a reward, and success in getting what you want depends on endless internal and external, known and unknown, factors.

Authentic liking, which serves you, your family, and your society, is beneficial for the collective life in the long run, and pseudoliking (for example, experienced liking in substance abuse or greed) is just a mirage. We will discuss why pursuing a purpose for your life (not an obsessive desire for pleasure only) is the best way to generate authentic happiness.

Liking a reward is easy when getting it is easy, will be delayed when it demands complicated cognitive and physical action, can be compromised by unruly desires, and is not always possible.

Exceptional liking cannot be felt frequently, and even if you are able to feel the usual pleasure from an easily available reward, or immense pleasure from an unprecedented reward, the next step in the cycle of desire generally ensures that your happiness does not last.

HABITUATION OF THE REWARD

All the best things in life feel great for the first time, but in time, their greatness starts to fade, and this is the most silent, tragic, and brutal fact of life.

We usually do not feel grateful and happy for the magnificent things we already have in life, but we can easily live in an illusion of elegant and glittering happiness from another reward in the future, forgetting that it will also become insignificant with time.

To completely ignore all the glorious and the most important things in life is typical human behavior in the modern world, and to feel miserable for nonessential and worthless things has become fashionable.

It is easy and requires no cognitive effort to discard the positive and to focus completely on a few negatives, whereas feeling grateful for what we already have, and putting the positives and negatives of life in perspective, is neither simple nor obvious.

The neurons responsible for adding pleasure to experiences prefer not to fire with a reward that has been consumed many times recently. When people respond less to the same stimulus after repetition, it is called habituation; adaptation is when people adapt to a certain level of stimulus; and when a motivation to consume a reward, such as food, comes to an end after its consumption, this is called satiation.

In economics, it is called a diminishing marginal utility, and marketing executives know it as advertising wearout. For example, bodybuilders need to shock their muscles with a new workout from time to time because their bodies adapt to the old workout, making it ineffective.

In general, your brain keeps killing the pleasure you primarily seek in life. Why?

The human brain appears to have evolved in the wild, where new things may have presented both a threat and an opportunity at the same time, as compared to non-changing things; as a consequence, our brains are more sensitive to the new but not to the old and familiar.

Because food is fundamental for survival, the pleasure that you get from eating the same food should go down so that you feel full and do not overeat or look for another type of food for different nutrients. These reasons provide some probable insights into the origins of habituation.

Habituation can be controlled to a certain extent but may not be overridden completely. Frequent consumption of the reward, attention on consumption, simplicity of the stimulus, and strength of the stimulus accelerate habituation. Variety, a break from the consumption of the same reward, and inattention to consumption and cognitive load slow down habituation.

The simplest strategies to counter habituation are variety and a break from the same reward. It is not burdensome for you to take a break from the same food and to eat something different, but it is difficult to do the same with other vital things, such as where you work, where you live, and whom you live with.

Unfortunately, circuits of habituation usually always have a say, even when things are out of context, and these neural processes can often override your recently acquired intellectual capabilities. We cannot get happiness from the same things with ease, no matter how critical they are, even when we are intellectually aware of it.

The incoherence of neural circuits is chaotic and often leaves us in confusion and pain. The limbic system controls us, and the intellectual cerebral cortex may be completely useless at times, even when you consciously want to engage it with the highest possible effort and intellect.

The desire that starts from a motivation to approach a reward may end in a pleasurable experience with the consumption of a reward, but with time, cruel subconscious mental processes take those pleasures away, and you look for pleasure again but from a different reward.

THE HEDONIC TREADMILL

You cannot always experience happiness from the same stimulus that is habituated recently; hence, you try to find a new stimulus to feel happy again, as if you are running on a hedonic treadmill, but your run never seems to stop. Once habituation ensures that a reward cannot generate happiness, a new reward is needed, but the new reward also eventually loses its appeal.

Apart from habituation, there are several other reasons that influence your hedonic motivation.

Adaptation plays a role in the cycle of desire because people adapt to their success and happiness quickly. Adaptation to recent success and happiness sets a new normal, and people start to chase a higher standard. Because higher standards have no limits, the pursuit for more or better can go on forever.

When the economy grows and income rises with it, new desires emerge. This rise in aspiration can negate the initial positive effects of a rise in income and can ultimately lead to dissatisfaction.

Social comparison suggests that desires are not absolute because people compare their well-being to others. Such blind materialistic relative comparison could end when one becomes the richest person on earth, but habituation and satiation can eventually transform something extraordinary into something ordinary.

In general, wisdom seems to be a better approach for happiness than money, once survival is taken care of.

DESIRE REGULATION

To prevent the probable decline that can be caused by desires, you need desire regulation.

By regulating out-of-control illusory desires, you can feel good in the presence of crucial things (for example, food and family) that actually matter, and your gratitude in life can rise exponentially by knowing that you, too, are vulnerable to the unfortunate and yet you have been saved from most of it.

It is a recurrent theme of this book, and it always seems unreal, but if you cannot appreciate the presence of good (and the absence of bad), you will not enjoy what you desire for long. We generally focus on what we have but not on what is absent. Focusing on the presence and absence of good and bad paints a complete picture, which is not too bad for most.

Most crucial things in life do not seem to give any happiness at all, until they are about to be taken away, but delusions of desires can be disrupted with the flick of a switch if authentic necessities are threatened. For example, a financially rich person will happily give up all of his or her money for health, but a financially poor but otherwise healthy person may live in misery, thinking about financial luxury.

Looking for new experiences in the future is noble, but sacrificing the marvelous and fundamental gifts of life because of delusions of desires is tragic.

Desires can be illusory, irrelevant, and damaging, and your life can be torn apart by out-of-control desires as they infuse more confusion and complexity into an already complicated life. We will discuss why following a long-term subjective meaning or purpose for your life is a much better alternative to reacting to endless involuntary and transient desires.

PAIN

As close as they may seem, pain and pleasure are not on opposite ends of a spectrum. Feeling less than happy is not always a painful experience, and having no authentic pain in life usually does not give rise to happiness. Pain and pleasure are registered in different areas of the brain, and different mechanisms govern the way they influence our lives.

We have discussed how longing for pleasure can take you away from pleasure, and in this section we will discuss why an inability to endure pain takes you one step closer to perpetual pain.

Pain could be seen as either physical or psychological. Physical pain can be caused by an injury or illness, and psychological pain has many faces: betrayal, breakup, loneliness, rejection, failure, disappointment, shame, guilt, grief, frustration, stress, boredom, insult, anger, disgust, resentment, panic, depression, anxiety, various mental disorders, and so on. For the sake of simplicity, all kinds of ensuing negative emotions (real or illusory) are called pain in this book.

In general, pain is anything that you want to avoid, but physical and psychological pain are interestingly different, and emotional pain is not absolute.

A memory or imagination of physical pain cannot create real physical pain in the present, but bad memories or missed overrated opportunities of the past, and real or unreal fear of something in the future can trigger psychological pain in the present.

When you think about the past, emotional pain can arise from lingering unwanted memories or from inaccurate or irrational thoughts about pain or pleasure from your unfulfilled desires. When you think about the future, inevitable and foreseeable events or inaccurate hedonic simulations can each trigger psychological pain.

Sometimes you suffer in advance because of your imagination, sometimes you suffer again and again because of your memory, and most of the time you suffer when you do not need to!

All of us have bad memories of the past or trouble that is brewing for us in the future, and not one of us can find a way around it, but such real suffering is not boundless for most people, and not many are dying from hunger or disease in the modern world, when compared with the rest living in the poorest parts of the world.

Illusions and a purposeless life are the primary reasons for pain when there is no obvious biological reason. Illusions are unlikely to cause physical pain directly, but they can inflict significant psychological pain, and if left untreated, such delusional emotional pain may develop into new physical and mental conditions, and can even lead some people to die by suicide in the worst cases.

Unlike physical pain, emotional pain can be highly subjective. Some people facing challenges or psychological pain can turn bad into good by learning and developing psychological resilience, while the same situation might cause others to take a long dive into depression and mental disorders. For example, losing a romantic partner or a job can be overwhelmingly painful for some, but others can learn from it, brush it off, and go on with their lives, to find better jobs and partners. Such cognitive strength is usually developed not by shielding yourself from the pain but by exposing yourself to the new and uncertain, and becoming resilient along the way.

The ability to learn, and to use already learned cognitive skills, come face to face with the challenges of life and determine the intensity of the emotional pain you experience. If you face challenges matching your current skills, you feel happy and engaged, but when challenges cross the line of comfort, stress results, and prolonged stress can lead to depression or other mental disorders.

When current challenges are no match for your skills, looming boredom brings stress back into your life. We will discuss how purpose in your life can solve this problem of stress and boredom.

In general, psychical pain can be stopped by taking a pill, and injuries can be treated by advanced medical science, but there is no over-the-counter pill for an agonizing heartbreak.

The course of preventative and corrective action is rather obvious in the case of physical pain, but the choices are largely ambiguous when it comes to the prevention or management of psychological pain. Emotional pain can hugely impact the overall mental health, self-worth and well-being of individuals, but a non-chronic psychical pain does not have such effects.

Overall, psychological pain is much more prevalent and pervasive than physical pain. Furthermore, the root cause of physical pain is not personal, and the source of emotional pain is not always absolute.

We know that both positive and negative emotions are the feedback of real or imagined experience, but why are negative emotions (which we do not want) so common when positive ones (which we want) are not?

NEGATIVITY BIAS AND STRESS RESPONSE

As discussed before, the human brain as we know it is evolved in the wild. Primitive survival circuits evolved first and the cerebral cortex last. In general, primordial circuits are also more powerful than the cortex, and only when your survival circuits cannot detect any threat to your survival can they let you use your cortex with ease.

Primal emotions (exploration, play, fear, panic, aggression, lust, and care) emerge from the primordial neural circuits, not from the cerebral cortex; and similar ancient circuits can also be found in animals. You think and plan with your cortex, and ancient circuits take care of your internal biological systems (most of which are beyond your conscious control and make you respond immediately, with predefined behaviors, when a threat is perceived).

The primitive brain was tasked with finding food and potential partners—and, most importantly, with keeping an eye on predators lurking around in the bushes—with the best possible precision. Missing an opportunity to find food or a potential partner is all right; you can live without food for many days, and you do not need to reproduce all the time; but failure to pinpoint a predator can mean death. Therefore, your brain is too sensitive for negatives, and positives are often sacrificed for negatives.

It is of paramount importance to learn from your encounters with predators so that you do not make a near-fatal mistake again (after all, you cannot make a fatal mistake again), and for this reason negative confrontations are saved in your memory more vividly than the positives ones.

Overall, perception and memory (the encoding, storage and retrieval of information) of negatives is much more intense than that of positives, and this primeval bias is negativity bias.

In reality, things are not just black and white. There are shades of gray. Negativity bias may involuntarily force you to focus only on negatives, discounting all the positive things in life, but you can almost always find both good and bad—no matter where you go, where you work, or who you live with. Predominantly focusing on negatives (which can lead to psychological pain), with or without awareness of such behavior, is paradoxically counterproductive, because you want to avoid the pain in the first place.

As the information available in the present is used by your brain to reweave memories of the past and imagine the future, focusing only on negatives can potentially convert good memories into bad and force you to predict only a bad future.

Negativity bias combined with focusing illusion, filling-in tricks, and other cognitive illusions can paint your entire life with negativity. This is especially troubling when you go through tough times, and you may wrongly conclude that there is no hope left.

How unfortunate is that, when a catastrophe befalls you, your brain can make sure it does not leave your side. Your brain can be your worst enemy.

In addition to bombarding your consciousness with negative emotions, negativity bias can influence your decision-making. For example, loss aversion is your preference to avoid a loss over an equal amount of gain—for instance, a motivation to avoid a loss of one hundred dollars that is more powerful than the motivation to earn one hundred dollars. You might also keep investing additional resources to a sinking endeavor because of your past investments in it, leading to sunk-cost fallacy.

The motivation to experience a positive outcome is less powerful than a motivation to not experience a negative outcome. You may not approach a date or start a new business because of the fear of failure.

In the wild, when you see a predator, stress response kicks in, enabling you to fight or fly (or freeze) from the impending doom.

Hormonal changes and physiological responses started by a stress response allow you to react instantly to immediate life-threating situations. The changes include high blood pressure, heightened senses, narrowed focus, the release of blood sugar, and a faster heartbeat; and these adjustments prepare your muscular resources for a swift physical reaction of fight or flight.

Stress response is triggered by the sympathetic nervous system, and the parasympathetic nervous system brings it to an end when the threat disappears and you have survived.

The brains of our ancestors were designed to constantly look for predators in the wilderness, and to react instantly and automatically with stress response if, for instance, a tiger is spotted. Fast forward to when we arrive in the modern world, with the same brains, our brains are still searching for predators in the environment, even when there are none.

And when your brain cannot find any tigers lurking in the bushes and the alleys, it might turn a little and completely useless thing into a tiger, or in other words, into a matter of life and death. Such a stress response is an excellent example of the mistaken activation of a neural circuit by your imperfect nervous system.

There are several pathways of information transmission in your nervous system. The same information can reach primordial circuits first for quick action and cortex later for thinking and planning.

Cortical thinking is very slow (it can take years to solve a complex problem or come to a conclusion), whereas your mind and body react spontaneously with ancient circuits, without any cortical thinking, if a predator is perceived. It makes perfect sense in the wild, but in the modern world, not getting a new version of a phone can also be perceived as a threat.

You can decide, using your thinking, what is good and what is bad for you personally, or it can be decided for you by cultural factors; and once learned, such cognitions and the associated emotions can be activated automatically, without any discrimination.

For our ancestors, stress response was triggered once in a while with the sighting of a predator, but in the modern world it can be triggered even when we are lying safe in our warm beds. This unnecessary activation of stress response, because of negativity bias, accounts for various medical conditions and for cognitive decline. Stress response is designed to last for a short period of time, when physical danger is present. Ongoing stress without any immediate mortal threat can contribute to a range of health problems, including high blood pressure, heart disease, obesity, diabetes, depression, and anxiety.

Along with ancient circuits for fear and panic, you also have circuits for play and exploration that motivate you to explore the world with playfulness, and to find hidden potential and bring it to life.

Unknown is where all the potential lies, but predators in the wild also occupy the unknown territory. You live with the same nearly two-million-year-old brain in the modern world, where there are almost no predators, and in stable societies there is almost no threat to your life—even if you decide to wander into the unknown.

As ancient powerful parts of your brain can activate emotions of fear from the fearless events, they are also equipped to turn endless potential which exists in the unknown into a predator.

When you approach a person for a date or go for a job interview or try to start a new business or try to enlighten yourself, you often wander into unknown territory; and certainly there will be feedback on your errors or failures in the form of pain, but there are no predators, as some of your neural circuits keep trying to project. Awareness of this fact, can let you succeed ultimately, because failures are needed in success (for learning), and a failure is not a predator.

Fear of a metaphorical tiger puts us in survival mode and hijacks the higher executive functions that are unique to humans (for example the ability to plan, make decision, solve problems, reason, form abstractions, and exercise cognitive control as well as other cognitive capabilities). Dread of an illusory predator is also an enemy of creativity, which is needed to find a brand-new and diverse range of practical solutions for the complex problems of life.

As discussed before, the human brain was not designed all at once, and new features were added on top of old ones. The appearance or disappearance of biological traits or features like stress response takes thousands or millions of years to take effect.

Nails served their purpose in the wild, but they still keep growing, forcing us to frequently trim them. Just as we cannot turn off the growth of nails or hair, we cannot turn off stress response completely. We can, however, learn not to fear or panic unless there is an immediate threat to life and physical action is required, because that is what stress responses are designed for.

Cognitive interventions are often needed for a sane life, because some circuits in your brain can be activated in an insane way.

Negativity bias and stress response work automatically and silently, making your life miserable from the inside. Your novel intelligence can be easily hijacked by constantly running ancient and powerful survival circuits, and using it for your own benefit is not straightforward.

Survival is the supreme goal for the primal brain still living inside you; and your recently acquired intelligence, which can often be illusory, is also too lazy.

As it happens, your intellect prefers rest when irrationality wreaks havoc in your life. External factors play their role in bringing pain in life, but how unfortunate is the relentless emotional pain that comes from you internal emotional elements in the form of negativity bias and stress response.

A part of you wants to prevent the pain in life, whereas primitive circuits run on autopilot, inventing pain when there should be none. Pursuit of pain is usually the default, and apart from making your life miserable, such pursuit has costly cognitive repercussions, compromising your ability to minimize and manage pain.

Now we know the primary reason why negative emotions are in abundance and positive ones are not; but is pain necessary for life the way it is?

PAIN IS INEVITABLE

You do not want pain, but pain is essential for life, as of now. There are several reasons for the existence of pain, and some are introduced next.

Emotional Feedback
Physical pain is an indication that your body needs your attention, and psychological pain indicates that there is a problem that is not related to physical pain. Your body uses emotional pain to guide you through the social world; if you are in the wild, emotional pain allows you to react quickly to events carrying life-or-death significance.

You also experience psychological pain when there is too much order or too much chaos in your life, or when you are struggling to make sense of life, or when you do not get what you want in the short or long run. There are endless other subjective and objective reasons for psychological pain, but overall, pain suggests that you pay attention, think, act on problem, or come to a conclusion that the problem cannot be solved.

Pain is how your brain tells you that something is wrong. Pain cannot be turned off in life, because it is the fundamental feedback requirement for a mobile human being in space-time, who can think and learn with the feedback. Pain is a fundamental ingredient of human life, and as unwanted as it may be, you need it for continued existence. In general, pain prevents you from going on the wrong path, just as pleasure tells you that you are moving in the right direction according to your own subjective definition of right and wrong. There are common biological reasons for pain as well.

Negative emotions make you suffer, but you need them, because they allow you to function in the real world. However, an inability to verify the authenticity of the feedback and detach yourself from the pain once it is received can amplify your life's pain, making it way beyond bearable.

Like the rest of your brain, feedback mechanism of pain (and pleasure) is far from perfect and there are two fundamental problems. First, feedback can be fake or ambiguous; second, pain often sticks with you after the feedback is received.

Psychological pain can be delusional, and it usually sticks around even when it has outlived its use of providing feedback (as if emotional pain is the actual solution to the problem). For example, we have discussed how things not needed for survival are nice to have, but they cannot guarantee happiness. Therefore, any painful feedback you receive in such situations is usually fake; and you can live forever with such pain.

If the road that you tread for pleasure gives you pain without any biological or psychological reason then that path is questionable. Pain and pleasure are there to guide through your journey toward your long-term goals, but they themselves are not the end goals.

Illusions are discussed throughout the book, and psychological pain can be often illusory.

When you make an error or do not get what you want, you feel pain, and such pain can be a focal point of your consciousness for a long time; however, pain by itself is completely useless and counterproductive. You should detach yourself from pain, learn, think, and act again.

The ability to disconnect yourself from your negative emotions once the feedback is received is essential for you to learn from these emotions, and use them for your benefit. Emotions are the element of the motivation framework; they are not the end motivation. They are supposed to be temporary feedback for your cognitions to find a solution and act again. And negative emotions cannot be turned off.

Learning

Learning is discussed later, but you already know that it is not always comforting. Learning a new skill usually takes repeated conscious effort for a few weeks before it is mechanized, and the most critical information in life is often acquired through failure.

In general failure and mistakes are considered bad and have consequences in the social world, but they are usually prerequisites for learning or in any worthwhile endeavor.

Learning is one of the most sophisticated cognitive abilities, and it is generally not possible without some kind of psychological pain. Being a fool, failing, falling down and getting up and again and again: this is generally what the path to success or enlightenment looks like. Strength and success in life can only be achieved through pain, and such pain is much less than that caused by illusion or stagnation.

Success

To find a date or a job, start a business, or any other endeavor, you need to try new things, without making assumptions. For example, you may need to talk to as many people as you can (every person is unique, hence every interaction is new), apply for as many new jobs as possible, and approach as many new customers as possible. The negative emotions encountered during failure and rejection will always be the part of the process as you approach the unknown. You can either detach yourself from them immediately (or as soon as possible), learn, try again, and repeat until you get what you want, or give up too soon, or not even try because of the fear of failure or rejection.

The pain that you get from a rejection is how it is supposed to be; it is just feedback suggesting that you try again, learn, or try something new next time.

Your brain is limited. You cannot control, know, or learn everything in advance. As you wander into unknown terrain, almost everything is new. You need to master it. This mastery is achieved by learning, which requires feedback, and feedback is provided by pain and pleasure.

Pain is inevitable; however, if you can detach yourself from it, use it as a feedback, learn, and try again, then you fulfill the purpose of pain, and you can use the pain to fulfill the purpose of your life.

Discipline and Responsibility
The discomforts of discipline are needed for living an ordinary life, too—not just an enlightened one. Parents putting food on the table and raising children; soldiers going to war; entrepreneurs powering the economic world forward, most of them failing along the way; students going to classes that they hate: All experience some sort of sacrifice. Without pain, ordinary life is not possible.

Blessing in Disguise
Pain is undesirable and miserable, but it can be a blessing in disguise. Profound psychological pain has produced great thinkers. Physical pain might indicate the onset of a disease, and a timely treatment could cure it.

You do not know everything, and pain can be a great teacher. If you train yourself to detach from it as soon as possible and activate your intelligence to find solution, pain can help you to succeed by teaching you what you do not know yet.

Psychological pain is likely to be an indication that your subjective map of the world needs a revision. The more intense the pain is, more opportunity may be lurking for you underneath. When nothing in your life works, you may go underground for a long time as you grapple with the new reality; but in the end you will almost always come out with wisdom and powerful new strengths.

You have to literally kill some neural structures in your head to transform, and you are likely to feel pain because of it. A complete transformation is likely to be psychologically painful, maybe for a few months or years, but it leads to an enlightened self, and life after that is magnificent. Obstacles are often opportunities, as long as you are alive and functioning normally neurologically.

Psychological pain may be the finest gift for you, and it can make you wise and strong for rest of your life. It can be your best bet to make sense of world and live with peace, strength, and meaning later on. Extreme pain or unrest can result in the death of the old you and the arrival of a new you.

Fitness
Though pain is an integral but unwanted part of human life, what you can do is minimize it. Ironically, to minimize pain you voluntarily have to go through pain, which makes you physically and psychologically strong; and the pain of becoming strong is much less than the pain endured in being psychologically weak.

The prevention and management of emotional and physical pain requires psychological and physical fitness. Such fitness demands that you get active, mentally and physically, and become powerful in both areas. Cognitive and muscular workouts that help you to deal with pain are not painless, but the pain experienced during these workouts averts the abiding agony of looming disease or disability, both mental and physical.

Your physical and mental fitness reflect a cocktail of nature and nurture, or genes and lifestyle, among other known and unknowns. Regular physical exercise (cardiovascular, muscular, and stretching) reduces the risk of cardiovascular disease, type-two diabetes, metabolic syndrome, and some cancers, among other benefits. Muscular workouts keep your bones, joints, and muscles healthy, supporting mobility late in life, and cardiovascular exercise improves the blood-pumping ability of your heart, which supports the growth of new neurons (neurogenesis) is some parts of your brain. Physical exercise also helps you to maintain a healthy weight and a positive self-image.

Similarly, cognitive weightlifting reduces the chance of your cognitive abilities becoming progressively worse as you age and keeps you cognitively fit. Cognitive fitness in the form of heavy cognitive workouts (to experience the new, gain knowledge, and develop cognitive strength) is the primary strategy, and it also takes care of your physical health.

However, as good as they are, neither muscular nor neural workouts are free from pain. A cardiovascular or muscular workout is usually painful, and physical inactivity due to disliking the discomforts of exercise can elicit way too much misery of medical conditions, than that is needed for exercise; and same is true for the cognitive workouts.

Muscle gain in not possible without muscular pain, and for maximum muscle growth, heavy weights need to be lifted when muscles are in pain, after a brief continuous use, and you want to give up. Pushing through physical pain and barriers forces your body to add more muscle fibers so it can handle the heavy weights next time, making you physically stronger. As you get stronger, weights which were a challenge to you before become no match for your newly developed muscles.

Similarly, as you learn to tolerate psychological pain, particularly when you are experiencing intense psychological pain (real or illusory)—when you want to quit, but you move forward anyway—your cognitive strength for going through pain grows; and once such strength is developed, unsettling negative emotions come and go but do not disturb you too much.

The ability to withstand pain is a fundamental requirement for a mentally and physically healthy life, and cognitive and physical strength minimizes suffering. Suffering cannot be avoided, and being weak is not a great strategy for dealing with it.

There are times when you experience psychological pain, and you know it is irrational. You may want to stop it but cannot; or it comes back automatically after pausing for some time. As cognitive strength (or skill) comes from neural circuits, which take time to develop, you may need to keep living with such pain for a few days or weeks. But with time, your consistent efforts pay off, and you will be able to control all of your negative emotions easily.

You cannot become physically strong in one day, and same is true for developing new cognitive strength. The key is to not give up, take care of yourself, and learn to endure pain—real or irrational—just as you tolerate it during physical workouts. Strength, mental and physical, is developed with pain, not without it.

In general, it is highly unlikely that you can be physically or psychologically strong without leaving your comfort zone, unless you are awarded near perfect genes and an ideal environment. The path to health, bodily and mentally, is usually greeted with primary pain, and pain intolerance attracts secondary pain, which can be avoided in the first place.

Psychological pain may be worse and more widespread than physical pain, but the psychology of pain suggests that ordinary psychological pain can be prevented and managed with knowledge and cognitive strength, which are part of your cognitive fitness.

Duality

Duality and relativity may make your life difficult at times, but difficulty can also make it interesting.

Happiness may become easier to define when misery exists by its side. Giving people everything that they need only provides happiness for a few weeks. After that we usually feel engaged with a balance of both ends of duality.

Life is not possible without pain, and when you cannot tolerate the pain that it requires, you resist life itself. You may think that if somehow you can erase the pain of the past, life can be normal again; but you do not know or control everything, and there is always a need to learn in this ever-changing and uncertain world. Feedback in the form of pain is almost always a part of learning.

You may keep the same path or start fresh, but pain is always your companion, and therefore you must be able to detach yourself from pain as soon as you can, learn, and move on. It is not that pain in the past was necessarily good for you, or fair, but you cannot change the past. Whether it is real or imaginary, intense or usual, it is best to learn from pain and leave it behind. That is how you can minimize it or use it for your well-being.

Both pain and pleasure are supposed to be transitory forms of feedback, but pleasure is usually temporary, whereas pain often seems permanent.

Death, disease, disability, encounters with malevolence, and the like cause real pain, and they remind us of how little we know. The rest of the psychological pain you can use to learn and transcend without taking it seriously, because you can easily suffer in the absence of any real suffering.

ACCEPTING VULNERABILITY

Even with a great deal of effort, it is difficult to find a person who yearns for pain instead of pleasure. But it is not completely in the hands of an individual to avoid pain (real or illusory, controllable or out of your control) altogether. The duality of pain and pleasure is fact of human life. Even if pain is not preferred by you, you cannot hide from it—and you cannot change this fact. If you do not accept this fact you will suffer more than that is necessary.

When you resist the pain of the past, you suffer again and again from the same merciless memories as long as you live; and if you are not willing to accept the future as it unfolds, you feel pain in advance for things that may or may not happen.

When you are aware of your vulnerability (along with the utility of pain in learning and in success) and you accept it, painful memories of the past become less painful, uncertainties of the future become less fearful, and cognitive illusions and distortions become less delusional and have less negative emotional impact. By learning to acknowledge and tolerate the vulnerability and the pain that is destined for you, you can detract from the distress caused by it.

The ability to endure pain is a fundamental requirement for minimizing pain. Without it, in search of habituating happiness, you may become addicted to external things and experience a greater degree of pain in the long run.

A disgust for discomfort can guarantee enhanced and prolonged unhappiness and mental disorders. Neuroticism (feeling insecure, being sensitive to feedback, having anxious thoughts or fear in the absence of any danger, having a lack of self-esteem, experiencing mood swings, lasting aggressiveness, and worried states of mind) and anxious personality disorder can be your rewards when you cannot withstand pain in all of its colors. Pain intolerance makes ordinary stressors in the environment extremely stressful, creates fear in fearless events; and puts you at risk of depression and anxiety disorders.

It may be obvious to some that bad cannot be avoided entirely, but a few cognitive illusions may delude others into mistakenly concluding that they will not be subjected to the negatives of life. The illusion of unique invulnerability makes one wrongly assume that one is not susceptible to vulnerability, and this naive positive cognitive illusion can facilitate self-destructive and delusional behavior. For example, knowing that smoking is injurious to their heath, people start smoking anyway; and many of them believe that smoking cannot harm them, because they are uniquely invulnerable. Call it naivety or overconfidence in one's own thoughts. But in time people generally pay the price.

The illusion of control can make you overestimate the control you can exercise on the events of life, good or bad. A presumption that preventing all pain is possible and within your control is just an illusion. In reality, negative events and emotions can be neither avoided nor predicted accurately, which makes resilience strategies a must for your health, happiness, and success.

Confidence in your existence, taking care of yourself, and giving life a subjective purpose or meaning are required for a glittering life, but overconfidence in whatever comes to mind usually leads to misery and can be deadly in the worst case.

When people realize that, in reality, problems can never be avoided, they invest their time and energy in building problem-solving skills and eventually solving most of them rather than wishing problems never showed up, or that existing ones would disappear automatically.

Accepting problems that just do not go away also forces people to come up with problem-focused coping instead of emotion-focused ones. Emotion-focused coping involves trying to feel good when faced with a problem without targeting the source, whereas problem-focused coping is solving the problem itself or coming to a conclusion that the problem cannot be solved.

Emotion-focused coping can be used when there is nothing you can do, but when problems can be solved, not confronting problems head on, and keeping them alive, means extended pain, which can be avoided to start with.

Embracing the burdens of life motivates you to make use of psychological sense-making neural circuits, to give a subjective meaning to your being and redefine your philosophy. Accepting vulnerability, making sense of the world that you live in, and finding the meaning of your existence may be unpleasant initially, but they show the way to a new life in the long run.

Identifying a subjective meaning of the world and of your own existence is critical for your survival and success. This introduces long-term goals, which motivate you authentically. Focusing on distant but meaningful goals helps in restraining desires that are problematic, tempting, and impulsive—and in promoting behavior that is actually beneficial for you.

With physical pain, you cannot choose not to feel pain, but with psychological pain, between stimulus and response, you can make a choice. A physical injury will inflict pain in all, but an insult will not, because you may choose not to care what others are thinking about you. It may not be easy the first time, but with consistent effort and repetition, positive habits can be formed.

Success and happiness in life are not achieved with one skill but with a set of them. The skills needed to manage the complexities of life might change over time, and new skills can be developed on demand. However, the skills needed to solve the problems of life may not be obvious, and an ability to completely accept unavoidable pain is an example.

Once you've decided, acquiring new skill and changing old habits requires days of consistent, conscious cognitive struggle, which is not necessarily enjoyable. Being open to the discomfort of disciplined mental efforts opens the door for inclusion of new strengths and lifelong growth, which is usually needed for health and happiness in life.

Negative moods trigger a desire to improve one's current state, and desires can get out of control easily. Negative states of mind can ultimately undermine your long-term success by introducing self-control failures, overindulgence in immediate gratification, and cognitive inefficiency. A positive mood, however, brings long-term goals into awareness and makes you cognitively efficient. The ability to withstand pain is thus conducive to success as well.

The unusual idea of accepting vulnerability and pain voluntarily, and not being afraid of pain, is critical for your growth and triumph. Clearly, opening up to pain does not mean that you invite it or do nothing to alleviate it. The idea is to be resilient and adaptive to things that you cannot control, avoid, or change, and yet feel comfortable with discomforts.

COURAGE

Being vulnerable, voluntarily, to whatever life throws at you, requires courage.

Stress response can be activated automatically by your survival software, needlessly and regularly, adding more chaos to an already chaotic life. Illusions help in redundant revival of stress response, and you need courage to either prevent the stress response or keep it under control when it appears.

Courage can allow you to face changes and challenges head-on by initiating a challenge response: the activation of play and exploratory circuits instead of circuits of fear and panic. Challenge response can prevent or override the stress response; it triggers a positive psychological state, which assists you in using your cortical circuits to solve complex problems.

Controlling your primal circuits of fear and panic is one of the most important cognitive skills for living a better life, and the challenge response is the most effective way to deal with it, because the circuits of play and exploration are designed to overcome the circuits of fear and panic, and all four emotions are primal emotions.

Primeval negativity bias and stress responses are the primary sources of worthless pain in life, and courage—when used with purpose of life, awareness of illusions, and other things—can prevent or control most of your unnecessary suffering.

There is a lot of ambiguity in every day events of modern life. For example, there is no certain way to decide which job, partner, or purpose of life is going to be the best. Simulation or prediction ability of your brain is extremely limited and imperfect for the external infinite. No matter how much you try, you can never know the future in absolute detail. It is perceivable only when you are in it. And, in addition to the ambiguity, there are real challenges in life. You may also lose your job, business, health, partner, and so on.

When faced with an ambiguous or challenging event, your brain can do one of three things: initiate a stress response with the emotions of fear and panic, freeze you, or let you voluntarily face it as a challenge.

By default, your brain is likely to initiate a stress response or freeze you, because the primal neural circuits of fear and panic are more powerful and easier to activate than the rest of the cortical circuits. Survival is always the topmost priority of your nervous system, in the primeval world full of predators. In the wild, your main purpose is always not to die, and you are living with the same brain in the modern world.

However stress response and a mental freeze are likely to make the situation worse in the modern world, where you need to think in order to solve problems. Negative emotions are the feedback, and the solution is to think, solve a problem, and act, or just try again when there is nothing new to learn.

To perceive events as a challenge, you need to minimize the automatic activation of your limbic system; and for that you need to rely on a few well-designed cognitive shortcuts or heuristics:

- Fear or panic is needed for a physical fight or flight, or any other authentic immediate threat to life.
- Pain is the necessary feedback to activate thinking (to solve problems) or to try again, and negative emotions are not a matter of life and death always.
- Do not trust emotions (or cognitions) blindly, as they can be illusory.
- Potential can be found in the unknown, and exploring the unknown with playfulness is a great way to live life.
- Life is great already with a working brain and body, at least in the stable societies, and even if it is not, obsessive desire, fear, and panic will make the situation worse.

With these cognitive shortcuts you can keep your limbic system under control most of the time, and then you can easily activate the primal circuits of play and exploration, which are part of the challenge response. These circuits bring the positive emotions of hope and confidence into your consciousness instead of usually illusory emotions of fear and panic.

Voluntarily facing challenges opens up your nervous system for mastery and exploration as opposed to withdrawal; as you develop courage in one area, courage generalizes, and can be used in other areas as well. Generalization is an extremely important trick of your brain, which can generalize both good and bad things.

Usual challenges of life convert to nothing with the courage and bravery assists you in being persistent in the hardship that success requires. Your brain can blur your cortical cognitive clarity by illusory fear, even when you need it the most; however, courage can prevent or override the fear.

Fear and panic are the most prevalent emotions, because of the primeval survival circuits still running in your head, and courage (which can activate a challenge response) must be fostered to prevent or muddle through the illusory pain that they can produce.

Courage also assists you in contending with your real clashes with reality.

BEING EQUANIMOUS

Consciousness is transient, and one's state of mind keeps changing. A full life is full of diverse positive and negative states of mind. Pleasure, pain, and equanimity are divisible states of mind, and being equanimous is not distracting too much or for too long from cognitively controlled intellectual states of mind, regardless of pain or pleasure.

Being equanimous toward the dualities of life is a surprising strategy that is at variance with your primary hedonic motivation. It proposes that you should control your desire for pleasure, and that you should have the ability to tolerate pain. It also puts forward a proposition that you should treat pain and pleasure alike, and you should be able to detach yourself from both.

Without a doubt all this is utterly unusual and baffles the common sense. This strategy first recommends that we open up to the pain that we so dearly wanted to avoid in the first place and, second, proposes to control desires for pleasure that have paramount predominance over our lives. Being equanimous seems surprising at first, but the psychology of pain and pleasure that was presented in this chapter explains the practical utility and the brilliance of this strategy.

There is more than just pain and pleasure (or any other motivation) in this universe and beyond; equanimity is an ability to have an independent and detached thought about any abstraction (or idea), regardless of positive and negative emotions.

Your brain responds to the equanimous state of mind with positive emotions, without you begging for the presence of pleasure or the absence of pain. And such a steady state of mind can help you to deal the chaos.

Chaos can emerge at any time in life. If you are not prepared for it, you may unleash it upon yourself. Chaos brings confusion with it, and a confused state of mind cannot contend with complex challenges effectively. Cognitive clarity is your most valuable intellectual asset—one that not only prepares you for hell but also guides you through it.

As far as your subjective reality is concerned, emotions of pain and pleasure are indications that something is wrong or right. It is up to you then to think and do what is needed. Pain and pleasure are emotional feedback, not solutions. This distinction is almost always ambiguous and extremely hard to put into practice.

The solution is ability to think clearly and critically, with difficulty; this is what equanimity toward pain and pleasure aims to achieve, by distancing and detaching you from the duality of both positive and negative emotions.

We have discussed the fact that you cannot hide from inevitable pain to alleviate it, and that extensive desire (wanting) for pleasure can be delusional and miserable. What, then, is the reasoning behind treating pain and pleasure alike and having the ability to detach yourself from the happiness (liking) as well?

Good fortune either becomes habitual or withers away completely with time. Things such as family and social security provide some stability, but things and positive emotions are still temporary in this world.

If something positive that you like a lot disappears, pain will generally replace pleasure—maybe for days or years—and this negative state of mind can make you cognitively inefficient. You will struggle to replace what is gone, if it is complicated. The pain that you feel when that which was good is gone can be directly proportional to the greatness of the good. You can experience the positive richness of the good, until you can, but when it disappears, it can create an equally great miserable void in your life. A good can convert into a proportional bad in an instant, and because the brain is negatively biased, the resulting memory of combined experience can be utterly negative. In general, memories are usually created with peak and end moments of a series of experiences, and duration is ignored.

Overall, an episode of your life can be stored in your memory as entirely negative even when there were positive things in that period, and the intensity of negativity can be proportional to the positivity.

With equanimity you reap the positive rewards of your actions, but you are also prepared for the uncertainty and habituation associated with the pleasures. Being equanimous does not mean that you do not seek out the positive, but it suggests that you should also be able to detach yourself from it when the time comes and it disappears or becomes habitual—and take action with clarity of mind, to replace or feel grateful for it consciously, until it lasts.

Desire for pleasure and hatred of pain are not enough. Great things are stripped of their glamour by habituation; the unintentional scanning for bad things in the environment drizzles misery on your existence; and pain is needed in the form of feedback for survival, fitness, and success.

Your hedonic motivation is further obstructed by built-in ancient and novel neural circuits and illusions (objective and subjective). Some parts of your brain want peace and prosperity whereas other circuits invade your thinking, weaken your intellect, and create possibilities of unnecessary suffering.

Extensive desires for happiness and illusory emotions of fear and panic further fuel distortions in your head and can even lead to insanity where you act for your own destruction.

Happiness habituates, and running away from pain does not help. The search for happiness never ends, and delusions of desires create pain, not happiness.

Pain intolerance hinders physical and psychological growth, subverts your success, induces psychological pain from memory and illusory imagination, and makes you suffer more than that is unavoidable and necessary.

As peculiar as it may be, the more you try to experience happiness the more it eludes you, and the more you want to avoid pain the more you advance toward it.

Your desire to experience perpetual pleasure is adversary to pleasure itself, and your intolerance of pain promotes much more pain in life than that is destined for you. Therefore, not getting disturbed (too much) by the dualities of life is the best strategy to successfully deal with the primary yet paradoxical hedonic motivation.

The strategy of equanimity suggests that you become relatively unshakable and come back to an indifferent intellectual state of mind when diversion happens. It protects you from miserable delusions and the cognitive inefficiency of desire, and enables you to deal with undesirable.

Unshakable equanimity provides an underlying leadership built on courage and intellectual clarity that does not waver much in the face of the chaos and complexity of life.

Time and again you feel emotionally distressed without even knowing why, because not all subconscious thoughts leak into your consciousness. With equanimity you can withstand or discard unwanted thoughts intruding in your consciousness, and as discussed later, equanimity can brilliantly prevent you from learning miserable thoughts and behaviors in the first place.

Equanimity toward pain and pleasure prevents cognitive

illusions, subconscious processes, desires, and disgust from seizing control of your intellect and your clarity of mind. Without clarity of mind you cannot differentiate between good and bad, and when you cannot separate right from wrong you cannot be happy or successful.

Strategy of Equanimity is puzzling, but it is meticulously engineered, keeping unforgiving genes and the world in mind.

SELF-CONTROL AND DETACHMENT

Your mind is not always your friend, and it can be your worst enemy.

The mind can be cruel, and in addition to letting happiness habituate and misery magnify, it devises towering distress from the delusions of dualities; marinates your consciousness in diverse and destructive illusions, posing as truth; makes your recovery extremely hard when multiple catastrophes hit you at the same time; primes your thoughts and emotions from internal and external cues, without your awareness or permission; lets you experience unanticipated emotions, which make you wonder about their origins; is made up of several systems, which can drag you in different directions at the same time, creating internal chaos and confusion; can activate neural circuits in situations that they are not evolved or made for; is shaped by nature and nurture, usually in an unhelpful manner which requires intellectual intervention for reversal; and usually acquires self-defeating automatic behaviors, beliefs, desires, and habits from the living world, distancing you from reality and tranquility.

Enmity of the mind is deep-seated, and the war against it has to be fought at many fronts. Self-control is the vigor that engages your rational, conscious brain in that battle, bringing sanity and rationality back to the mind.

Thoughts can emerge in your consciousness without any exertion, but thoughts can be illusory, having no connection to reality whatsoever. You usually assume whatever you think, feel, or do, voluntarily or involuntarily, is beneficial for you, but the evidence that we have discussed suggests that automatic activity in the head can be reckless.

Focusing more on the downside of subjective behavior that you acquire from the civilization, this chapter presents further evidence to propose that your mind can act as your adversary, and exerting authority over your mind is a fundamental necessity for a thriving life that does not deceive itself.

We have already discussed a lot about the biological folly of the human brain, and more will follow, but your subjective behavior, which your nervous system has learned from your environment, can be equally disturbing.

In this chapter we will discuss the positive and negative aspects of learning, memory, two systems, nature, nurture and personality; the fallacies of cognitive distortions and subjective beliefs; and, finally, why you need self-control.

LEARNING

In general, you do not do everything that you do out of the blue; you do it because you have learned things from your past, and your genes have been learning for many millions of years. Learning is a set of divergent techniques and procedures, which produce a lasting change in you from your experiences with life.

Of the several ways to learn, the main classes are classical conditioning (also second-order conditioning and unconscious conditioning), operant conditioning, and observational learning.

Classical Conditioning

A stimulus is input from senses, and a specific stimulus (sight of food or blood) produces a particular response (salivation or fear) in you. Such endless associations make sense, and you wouldn't survive without them, but there is much more that your brain does in this regard that it probably should not.

For example, a soldier goes to a war, and fear of uncertain death is a natural response. But when the soldier is back home, the sound of a helicopter can generate similar anxiety if helicopters were used extensively in the war.

This kind of learning is called classical conditioning, where a neutral stimulus (the sound of a helicopter) generates the response of a natural stimulus (going to war) by itself after both are paired repeatedly. Classical conditioning can produce both positive and negative natural emotions, by totally irrelevant things, when there should be none.

If you have survived emotionally loaded, highly unpleasant times, your brain picks up inappropriate things that coexisted with the natural stimulus and associates the miserable response of the natural stimulus with the neutral stimulus. When the natural stimulus is gone, you can still suffer from the neutral stimulus.

Classical conditioning can make sure you suffer again and again, with the same miserable experience, by neutral things, even when the original pain is long gone.

Classical conditioning does not produce only negative emotions. Advertisers associate their products (neutral stimulus) with attractive models (natural stimulus), and products start generating the same positive emotions even in the absence of models.

You might try to figure out such kinds of classical conditioning in your life and try to fix the inappropriate relationships between a neutral stimulus and its irrational response, but it is much harder than you think. Once a neutral stimulus generates a natural response, it can behave like a natural stimulus and can create second-order conditioning. With generalization, several neutral stimuli similar to the first conditioned stimulus are capable of generating natural responses.

For example, in the case of the soldier discussed before, when the sound of a helicopter is paired with the sound of a bird, birds can cause the emotion of fear because of second-order conditioning; and the sound of a plane can also give rise to fearful emotions because of the generalization without pairing.

Second-order conditioning is one of the reasons some people value money more than the things it can buy. Money is usually used to buy gratifying objects, but it is a neutral stimulus. However, it often acts as a natural stimulus.

Your brain is capable of learning reliable and unreliable behaviors and can generate emotions which do not make any sense. Classical conditioning suggests that you cannot always trust emotions that pop up automatically in your head—especially when stakes are high, or when your automatic emotions make you suffer.

Positive and negative emotions can be evoked by classical conditioning, and perceptions of pain and pleasure play a role in the acquisition and extinction of classical conditioning.

The acquisition of classical conditioning happens when a neutral stimulus is paired with a natural stimulus, and you also have some expectations in your mind. For example, in the case of our soldier, it is the expectation of not dying that forms classical conditioning.

Extinction—when a neutral stimulus gradually loses its ability to produce a natural response—happens when it is not paired with the natural stimulus for a long time. However, extinction takes its own time, and to accelerate the extinction of associations between a neutral stimulus and a natural response, people are exposed repeatedly to their fears in safe settings. (This is called exposure therapy.)

As discussed earlier, desires, no matter how noble they may be, may have distressing consequences, and in trying to avoid pain, pain can be prolonged by your brain because of classical conditioning. The ability to endure pain helps in the extinction of the learned miserable classical conditioning you want to dispense with, and having minimum desires prevents such learning in the first place.

Being equanimous can help you in mysterious ways.

Neural, evolutionary and cognitive components create classical conditioning, and are subjected to all; but what you learn, or made to learn, is subjective to you. The reactive nature of classical conditioning installs behaviors in you that are outside of your awareness. Classical conditioning is involuntary, and you do not choose to make irrelevant associations between things and the responses; they are made for you inadvertently.

Careful reflection will reveal unwanted positive and negative emotions that arise automatically in your head, and you can take steps to wipe out such conditioned miserable responses.

Also, being equanimous helps you in managing expectations, preventing acquisitions, and in expediting extinctions.

Operant Conditioning

Operant conditioning is a kind of learning where punishment and reward determine whether a behavior is learned or not.

Some of your behaviors have some impact on the environment in which you operate, and if those behaviors are followed by the rewards, they are more likely to be repeated than those which lead to some kind of pain or punishment. Reward can be a pleasant experience or just relief from pain, and punishment can be the introduction of discomforts or the reduction of comforts.

For example, when kids, students, and employees behave in an obliging manner, they are rewarded with pocket money, good grades, and bonuses; and when behaviors are not acceptable, some kind of punishment (no pocket money and house chores, poor grades, and no bonus or firing) becomes the reward.

Punishment in various forms is prevalent in our schools, homes, and businesses; and for the most part, operant conditioning can compromise creativity, progress, and overall learning itself; and this is the first major problem posed by it.

Rewards reinforce behavior, and are called reinforcers; pain is a punisher, discouraging the behaviors that precede it. Biological needs such as food, shelter, and social connections are primary reinforcers; and secondary reinforcers or punishers can be endless (better materialistic things or psychological objects, for example) which have nothing to do with anything directly with the primary needs (at least after a certain relative socioeconomic state). Secondary reinforcers, too, define your behavior, and this can be troubling.

In the modern world, materialistic rewards or punishments are extremely popular, but they have no known limits and are fed to you by the economic engine. While it is important to have that engine running to keep the world going, problems arise when you unnecessarily suffer because of it.

Learning from operant conditioning is effective when the time difference between a behavior and its reward or punishment is minimum, and two problems are created by this.

First, time dependency promotes destructive behavior when a reward is available immediately after the behavior. For example, in the case of smoking or overeating, reward is available immediately but can lead to self-destruction.

Second, when a reward is not available immediately and the behavior seems punishing, people may not participate in such behaviors even when they are constructive. For example, taking care of physical or cognitive fitness is painful (but constructive) and is avoided by many.

First, operant conditioning, operating on rewards and punishments, can make you to learn what is not good for you easily. Second, it will make it harder for you to learn good behavior.

Your hedonic motivation can determine what you learn actively by operant conditioning, with your awareness. Equanimity toward things decouples you from the rewards and punishments and helps prevent the problems posed by the operant conditioning.

Being equanimous is a startling strategy, and it helps you in mysterious ways.

Rewards reinforce behavior, and they are better than punishments, because with rewards the desired behavior is obvious, but in case of punishment it is not. We will discuss how purpose of your life can generate an incentive reward, which is better than the probable consummatory rewards of materialism, and other temporary things.

Observational Learning

Mirror neurons in your brain enable you to copy others, and this kind of learning is called observational learning. However, what you learn from others by mirroring them may or may not be beneficial for you.

Observational learning is critical for your survival, as you learn skills and fundamental behaviors of a functional society quickly, by copying actions of others. There is nothing wrong in following the common code that shapes and supports a healthy society, but blindly imitating the cultural code can supplement life's chaotic complexity.

Some societies are free, industrious, and least corrupt, and mirroring the same strength of character is good for each individual of that society.

A society with truth, trust, and freedom is critical for your well-being, and such timeless principles should be respected; however, what you want in your life can be highly subjective, and blindly imitating others can undermine the highly positive perks of a functional society.

Observational learning diffusion chain keeps behavior of an

induvial alive, spreading it across generations, and today you may be doing something that someone did once, a thousand year ago, and you can easily find evidence of it around the world.

If all of your desires and disgusts are that of society, and if they make you suffer, then instead of indulging in indirect slavery, you are free to unlearn what you have learned, using a simple act of observation.

IMPLICIT AND EXPLICIT LEARNING

Learning of any kind that happens without your awareness is called implicit learning, and explicit learning requires your awareness and efforts. Learned skills and information in your implicit memory can be acquired automatically as you struggle with the stressors of life, and some skills are explicit before they become part of your implicit memory.

For example, you learn automatically not to feel happy from the same thing over and over again, regardless of its importance (habituation and adaptation); and learning to drive a car needs your awareness and efforts for a long time before it becomes relatively easy and automatic.

Explicit skills may not be easy to acquire, but they can negate the negative impact of implicit learning if you know what you need to learn and unlearn—and, most importantly, how. Once you have that information, you can use explicit learning to introduce new, desirable behaviors or habits and erase or manage undesirable ones.

Explicit learning often requires relatively immediate and unambiguous feedback on errors.

When you learn to drive a car, your every action is subject to mistakes, but the feedback on that is neither ambiguous nor late. You know immediately what went wrong and why, and in a matter of weeks, you learn to drive.

On the other hand, becoming a skilled captain of a large ship takes ages because, after an act of maneuvering the ship, any noticeable feedback comes after a long delay.

And when the feedback is available, but the difference between correlation (for example, in the summer, the demand for AC and the demand for ice cream go up and down together; these demands are correlated) and causation (summer causes both demands; demand for AC does not cause demand for ice cream or vice versa) is not clear, no amount of time is enough for learning until feedback cannot be interpreted in more than one way.

Learning a new explicit skill when automatic and unambiguous feedback are not available is a huge challenge. In such situations, self-awareness could provide feedback, and self-control enables you to practice. However, the demands that you put on yourself should be realistic, and you should not expect a new habit or skill to be formed in an instant.

The feedback loop must be positive and inspiring, no matter how many mistakes you make while learning. Discouraging and demoralizing feedback will make the process of explicit learning even more difficult.

Self-control disciplines you, despite the pain experienced in the process of learning; equanimity pushes you forward through all the failures and blunders, which are required for learning.

Your brain is an associative machine, and learning can create irrational or damaging associations automatically.

For example, your brain can associate a few temporary failures in one domain with a complete and permanent failure in all domains (generalization). Such a flawed association will have destructive and delusional authority over your life.

Illusory associations appear authentic, and without enough information and discipline, there seems no reason to be skeptical of, and such associations can activate negative emotions and self-defeating behavior automatically based on internal or external cues. Learning, which is a fabulous gift, then becomes a curse, and your mind becomes your own worst enemy.

Genes, evolution, school, society, family, friends, work, media, politicians, corporations, religions, and the rest all shape your internal reality, and much of it is implicit. Your ability to learn, implicitly or explicitly, is a revolutionary leap in the evolutionary time, but this strength is not a strength always.

What you have learned until now, with or without your awareness, may or may not be enough for your current goals; and not all goals are justifiable.

Unlearning learning; which causes misery in your life; and living in harmony with other life forms, for a common good; seems a rational and constructive strategy to live life; and you are always free to make a change.

SUBCONSCIOUS AND CONSCIOUS BRAIN

Although the highly complex accomplishments of your brain result from several systems (ancient and new, automated by genes and learned since birth) working side by side, the nervous system can be divided into two logical systems: a quick, autonomous subconscious system, and a slow, effortful conscious system.

The subconscious system is extremely fast and powerful, biased, impulsive, and self-regulating. It executes learned skills; generates feelings, perceptions, mental representations, intuitions and impressions; needs less or no conscious effort; compromises accuracy for speed and adaptability; is prone to predictable and systematic errors; jumps to conclusion and answers the easier question; resolves ambiguity, often arbitrarily; and directs other automatic cognitive processes of the brain.

The effortful conscious system, on the other hand, is slow, lazy, logical, rational, and reflective. It requires cognitive effort, memory, attention, and motivation.

The subconscious brain runs life-supporting systems and executes learned skills and behaviors quickly and automatically, without your conscious effort; the conscious brain gives rise to your intellectual thinking.

Your conscious brain may be responsible for your higher executive functions (emotional regulation, reasoning, decision-making, cognitive control, flexibility, cognitive restructuring, sequencing, planning, prioritization, execution, and others) but it is weak, lazy, and slow when compared with the super-powerful subconscious brain.

Overall, the conscious brain would not stand a chance against the powerful and fast unconscious brain in the important matters of life if not activated deliberately and regularly. You can live a normal, modern life of frequent stress or boredom without actively and heavily using your conscious brain. But to live happily and effectively in the face of all that life has to offer, engagement of the conscious brain (with its cognitive clarity intact) is a matter of the utmost importance.

Cognitive unconscious is a set of cognitive processes that generate your thoughts, emotions, and behaviors; but you cannot experience them directly. The information that you receive from your senses and memory is used by your unconscious mental processes, and your permission is not needed for the activation of automatic and bizarre behavior.

Your cognitions and emotions can be influenced by things in your environment that you do not actively and consciously perceive, although you can, if you focus on them, and this kind of unintended perception is called subliminal perception.

You do not necessarily need to think in order to have thoughts in your head. Thoughts can arise in the consciousness automatically. However, you can voluntary use thinking in order to change or control your default thoughts, within the limits placed by nature.

We have seen examples of visual and cognitive illusions, which automatically arise from your subconscious brain. However, even when you can use your conscious brain, cognitive accuracy may not be possible with cognitive ease.

To see both brains in action in a different way, answer the following question:

A bat and ball together cost $1.10
If bat costs one dollar more than the ball, then what is the cost of ball?

The answer ten cents comes to mind immediately, provided by your fast subconscious brain. But is it correct?

The correct answer can be calculated by two extremely simple math equations, one for each given condition. The two equations for the quick answer are:

$$1.00 + 0.10 = 1.10$$
$$1.00 - 0.10 = 0.90$$

For the answer to be ten cents, the first condition is met but the second is not.

Using your slow and lazy conscious brain you can compute the right answer, which is five cents—and the correct mathematical equations are:

$$1.05 + 0.05 = 1.10$$
$$1.05 - 0.05 = 1.00$$

A mathematical error of this sort cannot cause any trouble in your life, but other cognitive and emotional errors of your subconscious brain—and the laziness of your conscious brain—can. A few are discussed next.

As the name suggests, the subconscious brain is not consciously available to you, and its cognitive activity can create a state of confusion, dissonance, and ambivalence. For example, you start running away from a tiger first, only to realize that there is a tiger, a fraction of second later. You can act without thinking consciously and not all thinking is consciously available.

In the case of simple things, the ambiguity or confusion can be resolved easily, but in the modern world, most things are ambiguous (losing a romantic partner or a job, failing in an exam, not getting a new version of a phone or any other materialistic thing, and so on) because of the infinite amount of information and the limits of your nervous system.

What is known is comforting, and what is unknown is usually scary; but the known is also boring, and the unknown presents new opportunities. However, when what is known to you is disrupted, the opportunity may not be obvious in the moment, and your subconscious brain can resolve the ambiguity using any of its neural circuits, including those of fear and panic.

Fear and panic are the primary emotions in the wild (where your brain evolved). From the thalamus, sensory information reaches to amygdala first, and then goes to the cortex via fast and slow parallel pathways. The thalamus filters information coming from the senses (except smell) and further transmits it to rest of the brain. The amygdala is the emotional center of your brain, and the cortex is the center of your complex cognitive capabilities.

As information reaches the amygdala—before your cortex receives it—your subconscious brain can decide first if any object in the environment needs immediate attention, and later it can contemplate what the object is.

The cortical thinking of conscious brain is slow (it can take seconds or years), and your primal circuits do not always wait for the cortex. An action or emotion can be initiated immediately by your subconscious brain, as in the case of a predator attack.

The fact that emotion (fear) comes first and the interpretation of what caused that emotion (tiger) comes later suggests that people can be wrong about their feelings. This is because the interpretation of a feeling or emotion can be accomplished in many ways. And if an ambiguity is not resolved accurately by your conscious brain soon enough, the subconscious brain can interpret it as a predator (even when it can be an opportunity), or as any other thing that it may deem fit, using endless illusions and tricks, with fear in the forefront.

Fear is still a primary emotion in the modern world, because the neural circuits in your brain have not been fully upgraded for the absence of predators; and unfortunately your brain is equipped to convert the trivial issues of life into a matter of life or death.

It is not that losing a partner or job is always a good thing, but these events are certainly not going to kill you (as your subconscious brain's automatic physical and psychological response might suggest), and fear almost always makes the situation worse in the modern world.

The thoughts and emotions initiated by your subconscious brain can be fake, but the misery produced by them is real, and you may need courage to fight the fake, metaphorical tigers (or any other delusion) in your head.

Not everyone goes to an actual war, but we all may need to fight one inside our heads.

If you learn something in one domain or for a specific situation, your subconscious brain can generalize from it in different domains and situations in the present, and then keep on doing so in the future. For example, if your job demands that you make a highly complex and critical technical system more efficient and error-free, then your brain can generalize a need for efficiency in your job to the trivial matters of your life. Similarly, if you failed once, in one domain, your brain can generalize from that failure to all domains for rest of your life.

Your subconscious brain can execute what you have learned in an unproductive manner; however, generalization is not negative all the time, because strengths (equanimity and courage, for example) can also be generalized by your subconscious brain.

Learned perceptions, cognitions, emotions, and actions can be involuntary and quick, and the design of the brain and the limits of cognitive resources do not stop your subconscious brain from making a wrong judgement or distorting reality, instantly and automatically.

The subconscious brain is built for speed. It does not have enough memory and computing power to manage infinite information, and it can never create a subjective reality that is the same as the objective reality. Stunning speed is the hallmark of your subconscious brain, and accuracy is usually sacrificed. With utility, such blind speed can lead to disastrous side effects when what you have learned (implicitly or explicitly) is not enough or is not helpful.

Your automatic thoughts and behaviors result from your exposure to your culture, and primitive behaviors coded in your genes, beyond your direct voluntarily control, may or may not be in your best interest all the time, but your subconscious brain does not discriminate between learned or automatic, good or bad.

The subconscious brain executes what you have learned, no matter how irrational and illusory it may be. The sad example of this absurd execution is a suicide. No animal takes its own life, but humans die by suicide; and humans have sophisticated cerebral cortex.

In general, a suicide is almost always a product of objective and subjective illusions, which the subconscious brain can keep generating. Your conscious brain can prevent a suicide or any other self-destructive, miserable habit or behavior (for example smoking, drug addiction, a sedentary lifestyle, and so on), but its engagement in your daily struggle is complicated. The cognitive work needed to correct the course of absurd behavior is generally too much, and your conscious brain prefers rest.

Life can obviously be brutal at times, but it can also be made beautiful with cognitive effort. The subconscious brain can make you suffer, but if you train it by using your conscious brain, you can use its magnificent strengths, too.

No one can tell the magnificence you can add to your life if you learn to awaken your conscious brain often, and use it actively and heavily. A sleeping strength is of no use, and it makes no difference how sophisticated it is.

It is one of the recurrent themes of this book that you do not know what you can do until you define a long-term goal, commit to it completely, turn off or short-circuit delusional cognitive noise in your head, use your intellect, and start with courage. Reality will reveal itself when you are in it, not before. Your brain is much more powerful than you think—if only you can refocus its strength from illusions to a well-defined, subjective long-term moral goal, using the intellect of your conscious brain.

Learning from the psychological pain of failure is part of the process. The pain that you endure during progress and enlightenment makes you powerful and confident; and such essential pain is substantially less difficult than the illusory pain that can be inflicted by the arrogance and ignorance of illusions.

Your conscious brain can directly or indirectly control the subconscious brain to a great extent, but it can't do so all the time. Simple things may be controlled by the conscious brain immediately—for example, not eating trans fats, or going for a physical workout. But acquiring an advanced skill or breaking a bad habit (for example, the ability to keep both mind and body fit, or not smoking), takes time, efforts, intellectual information, cognitive clarity, discipline, and a tolerance for discomfort, among other things.

A change that is incredibly difficult usually cannot be initiated without enough objective information. Learning or unlearning becomes easier when you know how your brain changes itself, and turning off the miserable noise of illusions gives your conscious brain a chance to make a change.

For example, quitting smoking is easier when you prevent the meaningless, self-inflicted misery of delusions and know what actually matters in life. When you bring your endless desires or delusions under control, the relentless misery associated with them slowly ceases to exist, and when you give yourself a lifelong direction to work on a few fundamental, meaningful, and worthwhile goals, nihilism—a sense of boring sameness or confusion in life—starts to fade away.

As you take action toward your meaningful purpose, positive emotions are generated along the way naturally, and your strengths are prevented from scattering in infinite directions.

The withdrawal symptoms of addiction may disappear in an instant with the realization of truth; and if not, then equanimity, pain tolerance, and courage will make them extinct in a short period of time. Pain is usually part of any learning experience or change anyway, and the pain that you need to go through with the symptoms of substance withdrawal is beneficial for you in the long run. Such pain is short-lived and leads to positive new experiences when compared with the worthless, severe, and avoidable pain of addiction.

Being equanimous not only prevents addictions in the first place, as you do not wish to be happy all the time and are able to endure the inevitable suffering of life, but also helps in their extinction—allowing you to withstand the pain of substance withdrawal with courage.

With enough daily, conscious practice, a developed cognitive strength slowly becomes a routine, and your subconscious brain can activate it automatically. In this way, you can have huge indirect control over your unconscious brain.

Some primitive activities of the subconscious brain can never be turned off, such as stress response, negativity bias, classical conditioning, objective cognitive illusions, and others. However, the conscious brain can be used to develop cognitive skills, which prevent or numb activation of self-defeating neural circuits.

For example, equanimity, self-control, challenge response, relaxation response (a physical and psychological state whereby muscle are relaxed; breathing, blood pressure and heart rate are reduced; and cortical activity is suppressed), and other cognitive strengths can be used to minimize and manage stress response.

Equanimity will numb miserable delusions of desires, and prevent or manage inappropriate learning caused by classical and operant conditioning. Challenge response can prevent or override stress response. Relaxation response can be activated consciously, and it can bring stress response to an end. However, endless illusions must be brought under control by knowledge so that your conscious brain can deal with the finite and real.

You cannot have direct control over your subconscious brain and its imperfections all the time. Sometimes you can easily control it, and at other times it may take a few weeks before you learn new strengths and unlearn your weaknesses. Some circuits cannot be erased; however, they can be prevented from activation—or overridden once activated by the effective use of the conscious brain. One way or another you do have much freedom, and you can take responsibility for your own life and let it thrive.

Your subconscious or conscious brain can be your friend or your foe, depending on known and unknown factors. Using self-control you can train your subconscious brain to behave rationally and positively most of the time. You can never erase the hostility of your own brain but with self-control, you can limit it.

SINS OF MEMORY

Memory is the ability to encode (the transformation of your perceptions, thoughts, and emotions into storable neural memory), store, and retrieve information over time.

Just like a computer or any other electronic device, you have short-term and long-term memory, as we can see in figure 12.

Information comes to short-term memory from your senses, and from long-term memory by the retrieval of encoded and stored information. Your short-term memory can hold only a little amount of sensory and nonsensuous information for a limited time, and your focus can guide what you hold in it. Visual information is held for around one second, auditory information for nearly five seconds, and nonsensuous information for around fifteen seconds.

Your short-term memory needs rehearsal (repetition) or focus for the information not to get lost. For example, you can hold a phone number in your short-term memory for a few seconds, after which it will be lost without focus and repetition.

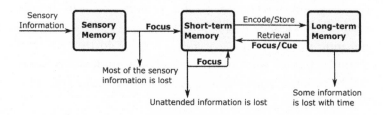

Figure 12
Memory

Information available in short-term memory can be moved to long-term memory with the help of encoding. Your long-term memory can store a huge amount of information, but it is also limited.

Your motivation and focus can influence encoding and storage, and cues can affect retrieval. For example, the phone number of a date is easier to hold in the short-term term memory and transfer to long-term memory because of your motivation and attention; and being in the same place where you met your date for the first time can help you to recall the phone number because of some external cues.

Focus influences your memory, and everything that you think, feel, and act upon arises from your memory. Focus is your most critical neural resource. We will discuss the need to control your focus later.

You can retrieve what has been encoded and stored in your long-term memory and bring it into your short-term memory; however, memory retrieval is also dependent on cues in the internal and external world.

A cue is the memory associated with a stored memory, and it can help bring the memory into your consciousness, consciously or unconsciously. A cue can be external or internal. The external physical place, and the internal psychological state at the time of encoding and storage of a specific memory, can help in easier recall. For example, a place where you go to drink with your romantic partner becomes a cue, and going to that place will remind you to call your partner for a drink, if you are still together, and be happy again. Otherwise such recall can make you sad or depressed.

Similarly, a happy memory is encoded and stored during a happy mental state, and as a result a pleasant state of mind can help in the recall of a pleasant memory.

Unfortunately, the same is true for sad memories. Your brain will help in the recall of painful memories when you are already in psychological pain, so that you can feel more pain in the present; and with filling in illusion, your brain can paint the pain over your entire future or past.

A cue can fill your consciousness with what you have learned, and it is not always beneficial for you. Self-control and knowledge can help you to change the contents of your consciousness, and equanimity and courage will help you to endure the pain while it lasts.

Long-term memory can be divided into implicit memory and explicit memory.

Implicit memory influences your behavior and thought via experiences in the past. Conscious recall is not needed for the activation of the learned behavior initiated from the implicit memory. Explicit memory lets you retrieve your past experiences, knowledge, facts, and abstractions consciously.

Implicit memory is the collection of procedural memory (cognitive and motor skills) and priming (perception enhanced by stimulus). Explicit memory is divided into episodic memory (your experiences) and semantic memory (your knowledge).

Cognitive fitness updates your procedural memory with cognitive strengths, and your semantic memory with advanced knowledge of internal and external worlds; activates, controls, or overrides priming according to cognitive strength and knowledge; and suggests that you experience the unknown for new potential or purpose of your life.

Your experiences, knowledge, and skills may or may not help you, and priming influences your consciousness from the cues without your awareness. Cognitive fitness can correct or update your memory for your benefit.

Some experiences can be unforgiving. Instead of numbing them, your brain may attach utter significance to them so that you can possibly suffer for your whole life with your memory, especially if you are pain-intolerant. Your knowledge or skills may be insufficient or too self-defeating for your purpose. There are ways to compensate for that: Read the great works of literature for knowledge and develop cognitive skills.

As you expose yourself to new experiences, gain knowledge, and become stronger, the practical utility of your overall memory rises. We have already discussed a lot about the importance of exploration, knowledge, and skills, and more will follow.

Priming is discussed next.

Priming is unconscious behavior or recall of implicit memory caused by a recent experience of a stimulus such as a word, object, or idea. For example, briefly holding a warm cup of coffee can make people to unconsciously believe that other people are generous and caring, and holding a cold cup of coffee has the opposite effect. Hearing or thinking about old age makes people to walk slowly (the ideomotor effect), and making people act old triggers thoughts of being old. The list goes on and on.

One stimulus or idea primes another behavior, memory, or idea and becomes a cue. The new cue further activates more cues, starting a cascade of activity in the brain. This activity happens without your awareness, and out of many active ideas in subconsciousness, only a few are registered in your consciousness.

You do not have complete control over your thoughts, emotions, and behaviors, and internal and environmental stimuli can prime you without your will. You can, however, use self-control to direct yourself, either on demand or as a part of disciplined self.

As you expand your memory with new experiences, knowledge, and skills, new thoughts and emotions too can be activated automatically, just as the old ones. In this way you can indirectly have some influence over priming.

Priming also suggests that your cognitions and emotions can be affected by your physical posture. Standing and sitting straight, keeping your shoulders back, and displaying positive and courageous facial expressions all prime you unconsciously and reward you with positive and confident emotions.

Your memory is not always your friend, but it can be made so by self-control, which can administer the memory by the exposure to the new experiences, primed thoughts and behavior, knowledge acquisition, and skill development.

The brain has its nature, and your nurture has an unparalleled influence on the way you perceive, think, feel and act. Now that we have a high level understanding of the nature of brain, interplay between nature and nurture is discussed next, with emphasis on nurture.

NATURE AND NURTURE

Nature is the biology of the brain, and nurture is the shaping of your nervous system by the environment. Nature defines the laws of brain function, which are common for all humans, and nurture is different for each of us, forcing a relative uniqueness in each one of us. Genes (part of nature) create your neural fabric, and the environment (nurture) fabricates the fabric of neurons.

Experiences and events, especially in early life, form and strengthen connections among neurons, and this wiring of neurons gives rise to a nervous system, which is heavily dominated by the environment. Even a tiny event can have a huge impact on the nervous system, and the wiring of neurons revolves around countless sequential series of inputs from the environment. Information in each moment is unlimited, and each one of us experiences a unique set of events in a unique sequence, resulting in a unique nervous system.

As discussed before, the primary motivation of the nervous system is supposed to be survival; however, thinking can control or override this primary motivation, forcing people to die by suicide at one extreme or to thrive at the other. Thinking can also make you live without any definite motivation, with nihilism, with chronic stress, or with pathological pain, and so on.

In general, what a nervous system can do is heavily dependent on thoughts, which are excessively influenced by nurture. Thoughts influence not only your motivation but also the other elements of the motivation framework: perceptions, actions (behaviors), and emotions.

The link between cognition and action (thought and behavior) is interesting. Action came before cognition in evolution. Single cell organism move, but they cannot think like us, and we seem to have evolved from them. You can also act without any thought, as you do when you touch a hot surface and your hand is retracted automatically.

Sometimes we act, but we cannot articulate the reason for action consciously, and animals can play a game without having any sophisticated thoughts of its rules. Cognition can obviously change how you act, but how you act can also change your cognitions by priming.

Nature and nurture can influence cognition and action together in an arbitrary or ambiguous manner, and because of this, thought and behavior are often coupled together.

We may have similar thoughts, but they cannot be exactly the same. Some environmental inputs are common and can lead to common behavior: language, clothing, social norms, religion, and the rest. Overall, two nervous systems may be similar, but they are always unique.

Where a person is born and lives decides much of his or her thought and behavior, and people in a given culture tend to think and behave in a similar fashion automatically. Nurture, among other things, casts the character, and most people of a culture have a resemblance in their character.

If identical twins (same genes) are raised since birth in two completely different societies, then, after reaching adulthood, their thoughts and behaviors (including desires, values, beliefs, habits and so on) are likely to resemble those of others in their societies.

Behaviors and thoughts can be learned from the environment during the early years of life without any conscious intellectual cognitive effort, and once formed, they run on autopilot, regardless of the associated utility or accuracy.

What is learned and grasped during the early years of life forms a subjective, simple, and limited map of the objective, complex, and infinite universe, and this personal map is critical for a person to make sense of the world.

It takes a long time and much effort to build a practical framework of incomprehensible reality, and we find solace in it, at least as long as it works. Any challenge to the subjective map is often seen as suspicious and subsequently discarded, even when its practical utility is questioned, and solvable problems remain unsolved.

A change in the subjective map of everything is not easy, because the world is too complex, and it is a huge intellectual work to redefine the internal meaning of everything known and unknown; and human brain has unlimited capacity to ignore its ignorance. There are several other factors.

Overconfidence is a fundamental feature of the brain, and it may or may not be productive. If what your think or do helps you, your family, and the community in the long run, overconfidence has its practical utility. But when it makes you suffer, it is clearly not a great strategy.

We have discussed the fact that arrogance and ignorance are the inherent nature of the brain, and they are often a stumbling block for an overhaul of the subjective sense of self. When presented with contradictory evidence, people with overconfident minds often strengthen their existing illusory beliefs with confirmation bias.

However, any voluntary practical and positive change is also resisted by the nervous system—first, because literally killing old learned neural circuits is painful and difficult; and second, because new neural circuits which can override or control old circuits take time, cognitive effort, and mistakes to develop, which is again painful.

It is one of the recurrent themes of this book that pain that you endure during a positive transformation of your personality may be intense at first, but it makes you stronger, more confident, and happier in the long run; just like the pain that you experience during physical exercise can reduce the dreadful pain of premature death, disease, and disability.

Your family, school, society, media, and the rest have sculpted your nervous system, and every major source of influence is likely to have its advantages and disadvantages. Parents and teachers may or may not know enough to deal with the complex challenges of life, and the media is infiltrated by economic and political propaganda, which is likely to be unhelpful in the most cases. Politics, economics, and religion are the major sources of influence on communities, families, schools, media, and individuals, and all have elements of imperfection that can be learned.

In general, a society shapes its people, and each society has different definitions of good and bad. However, some moral values seems to be common across all well-functioning societies, like trust, truth, freedom of speech, equality of opportunity (not the illusory equality of outcome; nature is never fair), civility, industriousness, and the like; and rest of the values are endless.

Societies have been evolving and fighting with each other for thousands of years, and most of them are corrupt and self-destructive. Society itself is maintained under the laws of nature, and Mother Nature can also be make you suffer.

Your survival depends on society, and not all societies are same, just as not all people are the same. Each biologically fit individual or society has the potential for both good and evil, and assuming that every person or society is the same is naive. What you learn from your society may or may not be for your own good.

A single brain is just too complex, and societies are a collection of brains. The implications of this fact are manifold.

We have discussed the fact that a human thought can be illusory, and social beliefs are not foolproof, either. Many people trust what they are told totally, but there are always some who question everything, for better or worse. No society or nation can be perfect, but if a culture is among the best in the whole world, it is the best that you can get at this moment, even if it is imperfect.

Just as utopian perfection cannot be achieved by any culture, social change or criticism of a highly evolved, civil, and truthful society should be done with extreme caution. The probability that a highly complex system, like a society, which is already functioning at its peak (imperfectly obviously), can be made any better is pretty thin. However, it can easily be made worse by a naive or corrupt intervention.

Cultural destruction by corruption is obvious, but even the most noble and yet naive causes, like helping others, can backfire when unnecessary help prevents their psychological growth or takes away their purpose of life. Overall, truth and trust, action and purpose, are the most important principles for allowing a society and an individual to flourish.

A functioning society where freedom and trust are paramount provides a platform for you to flourish, but society itself won't do the hard work for you, and it will not provide you with the information needed for your psychological growth and well-being.

Formal education, the media, and even some so-called scientific studies in social science all can be a source of political propaganda on the left or right—even in the most developed societies—and to find the information that facilitates your well-being and that of your society is all on you.

Things are pretty rough in corrupt and failed societies, and living a fulfilling life in such a nation can be extremely difficult if not impossible. Many of the corrupt, oppressive, and outdated societies in the world are conservative, whereas they should be open to change, and many highly evolved societies, undermining the utter complexity of the communities, are open for a naive change.

These days, a drastic change in stable societies is often led by selfish or arrogant people who do not know enough about the fragile and highly complex sustainability of a relatively less corrupt and free society. They often try to impose psychologically absurd and failed ideologies from the past that have killed millions, all in the name of a subjectively superior sense of morality.

What is working in a free and law-abiding society must be protected and respected, because it is the best that we have now after millions of years of evolution, suffering, and death.

As far as philosophy of life is concerned, if it is represented in the form of archetypal stories written and enhanced by the wise, across many generations, then those stories are likely to provide practical survival strategies to confront the suffering and evil of the world. Even if we are skeptical of these symbolic stories (where an archetypal hero stands up against suffering and malevolence with courage), they make sense to something subliminal inside us. After all, we watch movies, even when we know that they are not real.

The emergence of science has contributed to the confusion, and the death of philosophy for many. We have discussed nihilism before, and more on the meaning of life will be covered later.

Humility with respect to our human limitations is an adaptable and liberating belief. We need both philosophy and science for a thriving life. A belief that just one is sufficient is illusory, and philosophy may matter more than science in many cases.

Ideas and ideologies, which exist in all societies, are limitless, and not every idea or ideology is good for you, your family, and the life. Nature and nurture compel you to think and behave in a manner that is not likely to be advantageous and sympathetic by itself, and what you learn from society is usually inadequate to help you handle the suffering or stress of life.

If you do not know how a complex system works, you cannot fix it if it is broken—and your brain is the most complicated set of systems in the known biological world. If you do not know about the weaknesses and strengths of your brain, its weaknesses are likely to take over its strengths, and the results can be predictably miserable.

Society does not teach everyone about the objective and subjective worlds, but without a basic understanding of both it is extremely difficult to manage the complexity of internal and external worlds—especially if you struggle to find a place between order and chaos, or good and bad.

The problems of life will not disappear, but if you know how the world works, you do not fight an already lost battle, and if you have a basic understanding of how nature and nurture influence your nervous system and internal reality, you can manage objective imperfections and subjective deficiencies of the brain and ultimately solve solvable problems.

Information in this world is infinite, and the importance of the information that matters the most for health, happiness, and success cannot be stressed enough.

PERSONALITY

You are likely to also have your own specific nature or personality. Personality traits are divided in to the big five: openness, conscientiousness, extraversion, agreeableness, and neuroticism.

You may have one or more than one personality trait, and each personality has positives and negatives associated with it. Some personalities seem opposite to each other, and you can have such two traits at the same time, and they can try to pull you in different directions.

The primary traits of each personality are as follows (which also means that you are low in opposite temperaments).

- Openness: creativity, abstractions, ideas, imagination, intelligence, variety.
- Extraversion: social success, affectionateness.

- Conscientiousness: love of order and organization, sense of duty, self-discipline, disgust.
- Neuroticism: insecurity, anxiousness, worry, self-criticism, emotional instability.
- Agreeableness: cooperation, politeness, helping.

If you have a given trait, you are likely to not have the opposite, but usually, you need both in balance. For example, neuroticism might surface as concerns about your safety and security, but too much of it will make you suffer; creativity is great, but the probability of huge success in any creative endeavor is virtually zero; openness to the new is important, but not in a state of utter chaos, and some order is needed for openness; cooperation is critical, but so is competition, and if you are too agreeable, people can use you.

When in balance, openness and extraversion help you to transform and conscientiousness, agreeableness, and neuroticism provide stability.

Know that your personality is not everything that you can be, and you can learn the other side of the personality spectrum as well.

COGNITIVE DISTORTIONS

Depending on genetic predisposition, stressors, and environmental exposure, thinking can be highly distorted at times. Cognitive illusions are features of every human brain, just as rationality is, but for some, illusions prevail over rationality most of the time and may turn into distortions. For example, all of us can focus only on limited information at a given time, and as time passes we can bring other thoughts or information to the mind, but if a person cannot divert his or her focus from one aspect of any situation, for most of the time, a focusing illusion can become a cognitive distortion.

While illusion is a hallmark of intelligence itself, distortions can belong to a group of people or just an individual. For example, not all, but a few or a million can believe that the world is fair and predictable all the time. Such kinds of distortions usually depend on nurture, and they are certainly not characteristic of every nervous system.

Distortions generally do not help and often lead to depression and anxiety disorders. The most common cognitive distortions are discussed next. Providing a complete or detailed list is beyond the scope of this book.

Emotional Reasoning

Emotions are not always in your direct control. The subconscious brain can generate conflicting, negative, vague, and unreliable emotions at any time. You cannot use your emotions for reasoning. Instead, reasoning should be used to question emotions, using some concrete evidence.

For example, we have discussed the fact that the human brain is negatively biased, and if your consciousness is usually loaded with the negative emotions you cannot conclude that life is completely negative. Most of the negative emotions of the modern world are illusory anyway.

Sometimes emotions are authentic. For example, you may feel depressed by a rejection, but such feelings are almost always temporary and cannot be converted into a fact that you will always be rejected. Emotions, real or illusory, are usually temporary feelings based on emotional feedback, not the defining facts of your personality or the reality of the world.

After a failure, you may feel foolish, but it does not make you a fool forever. Before becoming an expert in any area, stumbling relentlessly is usual, and it is part of learning. A failure is the feedback of your cognitive or physical action, not a permanent fact of your character, and you are always free to learn and adapt accordingly. Care should be exercised when life is emotionally loaded, and it is better not to reason using only emotion.

Dichotomous Reasoning
Assuming that things are either good or bad, right or wrong, black or white, all or nothing, and there is no middle ground, and no shades of gray.

Life is complex and chaotic, and duality does exist; but its end points are not well defined. A person can never be in a rational state all the time, and a highly irrational person may have insights of intellect sometimes. In every moment or in any person, there is almost always something good, and you can also find the bad.

Also, each person plays several roles in multiple domains at multiple levels, and an imperfection in one domain at a particular level does not define the person. For example, a person is usually a son/daughter, parent, romantic partner/spouse, brother/sister, friend, learner, employee/entrepreneur, member of a society and a nation at the same time, and perfection in each role, at each level, is just impossible. Similarly, there are several domains and levels in the external world, and one's imperfections do not state the complete truth.

Dichotomous reasoning is absurd and is not a great strategy to deal with the multiple layers of existence.

Catastrophizing
Blowing a real or imaginary, event or situation, out of proportion, and turning it into a complete catastrophe.

Only a few things in life cause great damage. Living without a reliable supply of food, a betrayal, being lonely, or living with a chronic disease are a few examples, and the rest are just transient events of life, both positive and negative. Predicting only bad events and, as a result, thinking about abnormally painful emotions—and converting usual useless events of life into matters of life and death—is distorted and damaging at multiple levels.

The human brain can never predict the future and simulate experiences with absolute accuracy, always. Most of the time, the future can only reveal itself when you are in it, and at other times your pessimistic predictions can become a prophecy that fulfills itself.

Hope and humor are superior to the doom and gloom of catastrophizing, even when the trouble is real. Being weak is not likely to solve any difficult problem in your life.

Mind-Reading

Your brain tries to mimic others, to predict what is going on their heads, but you cannot read a person's mind accurately; and even when they tell you what they think, they may lie. Forget other minds; you can never be sure of your own mind and know with absolute certainty how and why thoughts and emotions are generated by your brain.

Personalization and Blaming

Criticizing yourself or others for things that you or they do not control or are not responsible for. For example, in a relationship, you may think that it is your job to make the other person happy and feel guilty when that does not happen; or you may think that the other person is supposed to make you happy and put the blame on someone else for your own inability to control your emotions.

It is hard to define what one can or cannot control when the thoughts, behaviors, and emotions of every person are controlled by nature, nurture, and the unknown. Some things are obviously not in your direct control, and some seem to be, and when there is no ambiguity, self-blame or blame is not rational.

Overgeneralization

A presumption that if something bad happens once, it will happen always, and may be true in all domains of life.

For example, after failing a test or getting rejected in a job interview, a belief that one can never pass that test or get a job again is distorted. Failures are fine, and nothing worthwhile in life can be achieved without them, and using one incident to draw an inference about one's whole life is absolutely absurd.

An episode of pain that is supposed to be temporary emotional feedback becomes pervasive and permanent by such distorted and disabling thinking.

Labeling is taking things out of context and permanently labeling yourself or others; hedonic distortions are focusing only on negatives, discounting all the positives, and possibly interpreting positives as negatives; and fortune-telling is thinking you can predict the future with absolute accuracy all the time.

The list of cognitive distortions goes on and on, because brain can believe in just about anything.

BELIEFS

A belief is something that you trust to be true, and the basis of your trust may or may not be rooted in empirical evidence.

Realistic yet optimistic beliefs help you in the usual struggle and hustle of life, whereas misguided, pessimistic, and illusory beliefs can have adverse and unfavorable consequences on your health, happiness, and success.

Flawed beliefs, which you can learn from your past, without your awareness or any shred of evidence, could be a great source of despair and disorders. Unrealistic beliefs become your subjective reality, and you are likely to suffer unnecessarily as you wait endlessly for the unreal to become real.

It is not possible to document all the beliefs, because mind can believe in anything of any kind, and evidence of that is crystal clear if you take a skeptical look. A few beliefs related to health, happiness, and success are discussed next.

Health

We have discussed the illusion of unique invulnerability and overconfidence before. Deluded by them, many people believe that they are uniquely immune to mental and physical, diseases and disability. In reality, however, almost everyone is required to take care of their mental and physical health, and a distorted belief can be the basis of several medical conditions.

Even if you have near perfect active genes and thriving environment, future is not easy to predict and prevention is always a superior strategy, as cure is not always possible.

Without your voluntary commitment to your mental and physical health, your fitness depends on randomness, and you will be exposed to all that life has, in the absence of any defense; and life by itself is not comforting, generally speaking.

Happiness

We have discussed a lot about pain and pleasure and your beliefs about both matters. If they match with psychological and neurological reality, you can do your best to control much of your happiness from the inside. And when that happens, you become cognitively efficient at attracting more happiness, even in the presence of real or illusory pain.

Pain and pleasure are almost always your companions no matter where you go, whom you live with, or where you work. Realistic beliefs can let the pain and pleasure guide you in your journey, and illusory beliefs can unleash eternal chaos.

A number of objective facts about happiness and sorrow have already been pointed out, and more will follow.

Success

A belief can fulfill itself to a certain extent in many domains. For example, a fake medicine consisting an inactive substance like sugar can trigger a real positive response in some cases, if you just believe that it will do so. A fake pill, shot, surgery, or any other treatment is called a placebo, and positive or negative response to a fake placebo treatment is called the placebo effect.

To determine if a new treatment is a really effective or not, scientists give new treatment to one group and a placebo to another (this group is unaware of the fact that the treatment is fake), and measure improvements. If the probability of relief for the people getting the real treatment on the trial is substantially higher than that of the people getting better because of a placebo, only then can the new remedy can be considered effective; otherwise it is just your belief that you are getting better, or your body healing itself, or something else.

The placebo effect shows that with a real treatment, a positive and optimistic outlook can also be helpful.

Along with your health, achieving success also relies on your personal beliefs, and your ability to succeed in what you try to do affects your health and happiness. If you think you can do something, the probability of your success rises—as long as you keep failing and learning. If you think you cannot, you have failed already.

Your beliefs can create a self-fulfilling prophecy, which is your inclination to behave in a way that is expected from you. For example, if you think you cannot succeed, then you do not take any action, and failure is inevitable. But the cause of failure is your belief, and it fulfills itself. Without a doubt, a belief is not enough for success, either, but a positive mindset provides a start.

In general, success requires experience, knowledge, and skills (technical and cognitive), among other things. However, your beliefs can direct you to or prevent you from exploring the unknown, gaining knowledge, and developing skills.

You may believe that you do not need to learn anything new, and it may work in some cases where your nature, nurture and luck are in a perfect order; but in other cases you must find new opportunities, acquire relevant knowledge, and advance your abilities.

Overconfidence, without any real learning (with failures), may not be enough to pass a difficult exam, find a date, or start a successful business.

You may label yourself as a loser because you failed in the past and assume that you can never be successful again. However, such lack of confidence can be overconfidence in your illusory beliefs.

In any worthwhile success, you cannot be a winner, without being a loser, and an illusory thought of superior abilities may not be enough for success, either. You can only know a little, and failure and learning are always part of the productive process. Gradual improvements every day can compound exponentially in the long run if you do not stop and keep learning.

Mistakes are usually punished in every branch of society, and a belief that mistakes must be avoided can undermine your problem-solving. For success, acceptance of a mistake is required, as long as same mistakes are not repeated when there is no need for them to be. In the development of a skill, same mistake often need to be repeated.

Clearly, a belief system that gives you permission to fail does not suggest careless behavior, but it is coming to a conclusion that learning from trial and error is essential for your success.

Lack of confidence can also be a misguided mindset that one is not intelligent enough, and it can lead to certain failure. While it is true that intelligence is dependent on nature and nurture, it is never the only factor in success. After intelligence, conscientiousness (hard work) and emotional stability are the most reliable predictors of your performance.

You can use self-control to control your attention and short-term memory, to effectively use your intelligence, and in being industrious and emotionally stable. With self-control, usual success in life is easy.

Luck is always needed for any huge success and a great mind, body and socioeconomic environment at birth, are the products of randomness.

It is a recurrent theme of this book, and you can never know what you can do until you try. There are endless subjective definitions of success, and positive and pragmatic beliefs can help you to define your success and be successful.

Some beliefs can cause pain in an individual in one society, whereas in some other society, somewhere in the world, it does not matter for anyone, and still a local irrational or outdated belief can be an intermittent source of pain.

Beliefs spell out your philosophy, and deluded or maladaptive beliefs are often sources of emotional pain in your life.

It is okay and worthwhile to follow others when it is good for you, society, and the earth, but when the outdated beliefs (which are accumulated through the history of humankind) become an enemy of your well-being and that of everyone else, carrying them on your shoulders becomes a burden which you must not carry.

The world is chaotic, but some hold the opposite belief, and when reality reveals itself, more chaos crops up. Distorted beliefs may be helpful on some occasions, but the presence of positive beliefs (and the absence of absurd beliefs) is productive in general.

Critical thinking is knowing what you see (or perceive, think) and what you do not see and create doubt in everything that you see. A belief that is not subjected to critical thinking has the potential to make your life difficult and dark. Your expectations and desires make a lens through which you see the world. It is easier to jump to conclusions than to doubt, and it takes no efforts to keep ignoring what you do not see.

Perceptual confirmation is the propensity to see what one expects to see; and for most, evidence may not matter because of belief bias, which is ignoring logical validity, reaching to conclusions, only if beliefs are believable. Confirmation bias is the tendency to seek, twist, and interpret evidence to fit into your existing beliefs, even if available evidence is contradictory or insufficient to come to a conclusion.

Beliefs are easy to acquire, but it is not easy to leave them behind, even when they make you suffer. Once set, beliefs run on autopilot, and many of them may be controlling and holding you back from the inside, even when things outside are fairly favorable. Only a few distorted beliefs are discussed in this section and you are free to find out any blind beliefs living in your head, forcing you to carry a pathological baggage of irrational ideas which you should dispense with.

Life is not fair, but as long as you have physical and mental independence, living life to its full extent is not far-fetched with positive and yet realistic beliefs.

COGNITIVE BEHAVIORAL THERAPY

Behavior therapy focuses on changing learned behavior using the principles of learning—for example, using reinforcement and punishment derived from the operant conditioning in promoting desired behavior or eliminating unwanted behavior.

The extinction of learned behavior that was acquired by classical conditioning is also possible with exposure therapy— exposing yourself to things that you fear, slowly, and becoming courageous and strong in the process, which is part of behavior therapy. Cognitive therapy is recognizing and correcting distorted thinking about the internal and external world.

Cognitive Behavioral Therapy (CBT) aims to change your behavior and correct your distorted thinking by using strategies from both cognitive and behavior therapies.

CBT can be as effective as medication in treating mental disorders, without any side effects. If you have access to mental health professionals, then good for you, but even if such access is restricted, you can control your own thought and behavior with cognitive fitness.

Whatever the case may be, you have to do most of the psychological weightlifting (experiencing the new, educating yourself, and developing cognitive strengths) by yourself.

DETACHMENT

The fundamental error that causes relentless misery in life is putting complete trust in thoughts and emotions arising in the head, as if everything automatically bombarding your consciousness is authentic and helpful.

Irrationality and intelligence coexist in your head and can compete with each other, and detachment from both can help you in realizing the difference, which is not always transparent or obvious. Detachment, or cognitive defusion, is the ability to look at your own cognitions and emotions, in a manner that logical validity of them is judged before they are believed and acted upon.

We have discussed that your brain often assigns a lightning-quick, believable meaning to whatever it can manage, and accuracy is usually sidelined in favor of speed. Your cognitions and emotions are far from flawless, because they cannot be quick and accurate at the same time, all the time, with limited neural resources; and emotions provide feedback on your current mental and physical state, and emotions are often overrated or inaccurate.

Also, emotions are not the solution.

A complex problem can be solved by clear and critical thinking that can correct itself. Mistakes will be made and emotional feedback will be provided again and again, forever. Without an ability to detach yourself from your cognitions and emotions, complex problems are unlikely to be solved.

Too much confidence in self-activating contents of your consciousness can be a bliss; but not always, especially when you contend with the complex problems. If your life is good, as of today, then you can live with the overconfidence, without any immediate side effects, at least on you, and at least for some time; but uncertainty and change are woven in the fabric of space-time. The edge of the abyss is always present, and one can be on the other side in an instant.

Cognitively defusing detrimental and deluding thoughts and emotions, and infusing intellectual clarity in your consciousness, is the backbone of a life that is not the enemy of itself.

THE CASE FOR SELF-CONTROL

Although nature and nurture provide a platform for the positive and negative emotions to exist, there are so many ways for the corruption of consciousness by the arrogance and illusions, than there are ways for the elevation of exceptionally difficult happiness.

Startling cognitive illusions, biases, and distortions; vexing and disruptive wanting; heuristics answering easier questions; habituating happiness and the hedonic treadmill; erratic emotional feedback; real and regular fear of unreal predators from minor discomforts; internal or external cues priming your thoughts and behavior; destructive learning from nurture; sins of memory; mirroring others blindly; physiology silently affecting cognition; biology of belief and blind beliefs; a powerful subconscious brain beyond your awareness and direct control; self-defeating generalization of learned behavior; random resolution of ambiguity; things decaying on their own accord because of entropy; and mental shotgun and the transient consciousness—all these fuel self-deceptive and miserable emotions (and cognitions) from the inside and call for self-control to engage your intellect in a brutal war against absurdity and misery on various fronts.

Self-control is the primary cognition that can administer other cognitions (as well as emotions and actions).

Self-control should be put to work primarily in controlling the most rampantly irrational or miserable behavior at first (for example in controlling an overreacting limbic system), and as you grow stronger, trivial behaviors can be controlled with ease as your strengths generalize.

Internal or external cues trigger tempting desires, want-should conflicts, and need for instant gratification. As cues can be subliminal and cannot be controlled completely, self-control is crucial in the regulation, inhibition, and overriding of problematic desires.

Self-control blunts out-of-control desires and prohibits the behavior associated with them; promotes high pain tolerance and better cognitive performance; helps in the avoidance of emotion focused coping; and prevents indulgence in substance abuse and aggressive behavior.

People high is trait Self-Control and have higher intelligence too, because of their ability to control cognition, attention and emotion.

Building self-control starts with a belief that you can eventually control your mind, no matter how hard or painful it is initially, and then arises the need of relentless cognitive efforts to intercept and control your thoughts, behaviors and emotions. Subjective distorted thoughts and behaviors can be brought under control with efforts; but common cognitive illusions, and other unhelpful neural circuits can never be erased from your head, and hence self-control is not simple.

Self-control is also a limited cognitive resource and often needs rest.

As far as thoughts are concerned, thought suppression backfires and ironically fills your consciousness with the same thoughts that you want to suppress in the first place. So instead of trying to suppress your distressing thoughts, you should spend your time and energy in developing alternative thoughts (for example, making sense of the objective and subjective world), and until then, learn to tolerate the pain associated with the thoughts that you do not wish to have.

Muscles can be developed with painful muscular workouts and, once developed, require lifelong muscular activity for maintenance. In similar fashion, developing self-control (or any other psychological skill) takes time, effort and pain; and regular practice is required for the continuation.

It is hard to say exactly how long it takes to form a new powerful habit, but with enough recurrent daily practice, usually a month of self-disciplined and consistent cognitive exertions are required, which are likely to be painful. However, the pain endured in becoming cognitively fit is nothing as compared to the pain induced by illusions.

The most effective time to build a muscle is not when the workout is in an easy phase but at those moments when you go through surging pain. Your muscles are completely exhausted, and you want to give up, but you push yourself anyway for a few more moments.

Likewise, to strengthen your psychological muscles (neural circuits), you must fight unwanted thoughts in your head (to develop new neural circuits), no matter how much excruciating psychological pain you experience.

This fight makes new neural circuits for new thoughts stronger with time; and with enough practice, new cognitions can finally control or override the old ones. And the pain that you experience in this fight can be from the literal death of some of your old neural circuits.

Sometimes pain is authentic and sometimes it is a sham, but pushing through pain makes you psychologically strong. Life is not easy for most, and cognitive strength is your best bet to live with sanity and joy. Pain will be there anyway, and pain suffered during a positive psychological transformation brings down overall pain in life, and such transformation also assists in living a transcendent life.

At first, super-massive cognitive efforts to control your mind may be met with consistent failure, and you may also feel the pain of the realization of out-of-control illusions in your head, but this kind of pain is temporary. A mind that is not in your control generates psychological pain anyway, and you are free to convert the short-term psychological pain (which you endure during building self-control into one of the most powerful psychological skills that you can have.

Intelligence is imperfect. Intellect is liberating and marvelous but imperfections open door for enslavement and suffering. The higher-level intelligence of your conscious brain is lazy and weak when compared with the lower-level intelligence of your swift and powerful subconscious brain.

Without any intellectual interference, the subconscious brain generally has the last word, which in many cases can be insane. Self-control can however engage and employ your conscious brain to conquer inherent irrational or illusory cognitions, emotions, and actions, and bring cognitive clarity and sanity back into your life.

Waking up in the morning is easy, and any real cognitive hustle is not needed for a default thought, emotion, or behavior, but awakening your sleeping intellect to exert rational conscious cognitive control over yourself in order to solve complex problems of life is neither default nor easy.

Your intelligence may not necessarily come to your aid by itself as you face unforgiving challenges of life. The subconscious brain governs most of your cognitions, actions, and emotions, but it does not differentiate between good and bad. It just executes whatever you and your genes have learned.

Nature and nurture, pain and pleasure, thoughts and emotions, beliefs and behaviors, motivation and memory—all these can work against you, sculpting your subconscious brain with or without your awareness while your intellectual, conscious brain keeps dozing off.

The mind can easily be your enemy, crippling the probability of your success and subverting your happiness; but, with self-control, the mind can be disciplined with grueling practice and detachment, no matter how hard it may seem initially.

Self-control is one of the primary strategies for dealing with the chaos and complexity of life and the hostility of your own brain.

ACT FOR A PURPOSE, NOT REWARDS

Psychology of action, laziness, purpose (motivation or meaning), and cognitive efficiency, which is introduced in this chapter, suggests that you should occupy yourself with action, which gives a purpose to your existence; and yet the objective of each of your actions should not be a reward.

LAZINESS

Life evolved in the wilderness, where food was usually scarce, and as both physical and cognitive efforts demand energy, which comes from hard-to-find food, laziness is preferred to unnecessary action. Laziness is encoded in your genes, and it became an evolutionary instinct long ago; but in modern world, where food is usually available easily and problems may be extremely difficult to solve, physical and mental laziness does not serve its original purpose and is utterly problematic.

A sedentary lifestyle has been linked to many major but preventable medical conditions, and a lack of intellectual exertion can make you suffer relentlessly, which can cause additional chronic conditions. Inherited ancient instincts have made us predisposed to avoid unnecessary exertion for the conservation of energy, but this deep-rooted affinity to laziness is now not needed and destructive.

Regardless of the fundamental need of action, to survive or thrive, your body and mind usually prefer laziness over action; and as discussed later, the biology of the brain can further downgrade the efficiency of cognitive actions, which you are able to take anyway.

Intrinsic laziness prevents the awakening of your conscious brain, and mental activity is usually much harder than physical labor. However, cognitive action is what you need to conquer the deception and hostility of your own brain, solve problems, prevent preventable suffering, and thrive.

Taking action can be your conscious choice, and a proclivity for hard work needs to be adopted for a rejuvenating, full life.

TAKE ACTION FOR A PURPOSE

Several hedonic hotspots activating at the same time is a highly unlikely event, and it makes feelings of bliss relatively rare. Habituation further makes sure that your bliss disappears soon, if it even appears.

You cannot expect a blissful experience all the time, and still you need the motivation of desires to engage in life; but desires often lead to your decline, and if not a desire for pleasure, then what should be the reason of your any action?

It turns out that finding a purpose (meaning or reason) for your life and taking action in accordance with it is superior to reacting to endless transient desires.

There are several psychological, neurological, and philosophical reasons why a covenant that you make with your being, and taking action to realize it, changes the way your nervous system works in a positive way, and a few are discussed next.

Motivation

Your brain has a purpose, and it is to let you pursue your purpose in space-time.

The sea squirt starts off with a brain, but when it attaches itself to a rock, its brain is absorbed by its body. The brain of the sea squirt is made for physical action in the sea, and when action is no longer required, the brain also disappears. Plants are alive but do not move and hence need no brain either.

Your brain is a goal-oriented machine, and it is made for action in the fabric of space and time, along with other known and unknowns reasons.

As pointed out earlier, goal and action are the part of the motivation framework, which also includes perception, cognition, and emotion. In general, motivation sets a goal in space-time (usually for a better future); perceptions enable you to move in space-time; thinking can solve problems, and direct physical action; and emotions provide the feedback (real or illusory) of your real or simulated cognitive and physical action.

Everything that you perceive, think, do, or feel revolves around a series of goals in the space-time as you try to move from a bad present to good future in the space-time (or in your mind with your imagination), with hope, and managing this movement is the primary purpose of your brain.

We have discussed that the imperfections and illusions of your brain can make you suffer without any apparent reason, and a purpose for your life seems to be the only known strategy that can bring some order to such internal chaos.

The motivation framework and its elements (cognitions and emotions) may not let you live in peace if they are not directed toward a purpose.

Without a purpose your cognitions have no moral hierarchy or leadership, and your emotions are likely to be governed by the primeval circuits of fear and panic or by randomness. With a purpose of your life, whole the motivation framework serves its own purpose, and without it, everything about it can become your enemy. And your brain usually lets you know by making you suffer in the absence of any purpose.

Your cognitions and emotions are your friends when cognitions decide a path and work to help you tread it, and emotions guide you on that path with the emotional feedback. Without leadership, both cognitions and emotions can easily be your enemy.

In general, there are two fundamental motivations: to survive and to thrive. But survival in the modern world is not as easy as it seems with an outdated two-million-year-old brain. If survival is your only motivation, then your primal brain can activate a stress response (which is primarily associated with survival) and other misery-producing circuits frequently, in an arbitrary manner. Your cortex can control the primal circuits, but it needs leadership that assists in your survival and also guides you when your survival is not on the line.

Your decision to thrive forces you to find a focal point in life, and this focal point can provide leadership to your cortex in the infinite cosmos. As a result of deciding on a direction in life, your cortical circuits are likely to act in coherence and prevent or override the activation of primal circuits.

And what you learn when you want to thrive makes the goal of survival extremely easy.

Survival is same for everyone (eat and reproduce) and your purpose defines how you want to thrive in the real world. Your purpose gives your brain a goal to orient itself. Your brain and body can take you from a problematic present to a better future, but first you must decide what it is for you.

Motivated action is one of the fundamental needs of your nervous system, and without it, your happiness or prosperity is in the hands of randomness, and the outcome is generally not great. Purpose in life gives your brain a never-ending series of meaningful actions, and it saves you from the possible horrors of inaction.

Infinite Directions

There are several archaic and novel neural circuits in your head, which usually pull you in different directions, creating internal confusion and chaos; and there are infinite directions in the outer world as well.

Your brain has its strengths, but they are limited; and your cognitive strengths must be focused on something finite, for any worthwhile use; whereas the weaknesses of brain can be triggered in infinite ways. The information in the universe is infinite, and bounded strengths of your brain are of almost no justifiable use if they are distracted in an eternal confusion by internal battles (of neural circuits) and external chaos.

A lifelong moral goal provides pivotal leadership to several internal neural systems, competing for dominance, and a course for your goal-oriented brain to chart the external space-time.

Out of infinite directions in the external world, you need a definite direction in such a way that positive parts of your brain can come together and help you to move in a positive direction, whereas a directionless life is likely to be dominated by negativity.

Known and Unknown

There are a few explanations for the needs of left and right cerebral hemispheres, and an interesting one is: The left hemisphere is made for the explored and known world, and the right hemisphere tries to manage the unexplored and unknown territory.

It makes sense, because you know a little, and there are infinite things you do not know; and what you know today may not be enough tomorrow, when the unknown reveals itself. At the same time you cannot disrupt everything you know when you deal with the unknown. The separation of concerns seems to be a necessity of a working nervous system, and it can be done by letting each hemisphere specialize in one domain.

As far as pain and pleasure are concerned, both the known and the unknown can be comforting as well as discomforting.

Uncertainty about a job (or business), romantic partner, health, and other socioeconomic concerns, at the same time, can be just too miserable to deal with. However, the unknown in a little dose is exciting, as in the case of a new movie or music or opportunity. The known in the form of the security of home and family is comforting, but you do not watch the same movie over and over again, and you do not listen to the same music all the time. You need something new occasionally, which you find in the unknown.

However, the known and the unknown can lead to pain and pleasure in a complicated and ambiguous manner, and to live optimally, you need to live on a fine line between the known and the unknown. Your purpose of life can help you to deal with them both, if the purpose is difficult enough.

In general, if you wish to thrive, there is always a new opportunity or something unknown that can excite you; and the cognitive strengths needed to thrive provide you with an underlying known map of everything (including strategies to deal with the unknown or mystery of the universe) for some emotional stability.

Finding a balance between known and unknown is possible when you chase something difficult and meaningful.

A New World

When you move forward toward something difficult, the world is not the same as it was before and neither are you. You cannot simulate the new world in your head with your limited short-term memory, which lasts for a few seconds, and limited computing power. It awaits you in the unknown, and it will reveal itself only when you step into it, not before.

Perceptions and cognitions are limited and biased and are often dependent on your focus, which can be directed by your purpose. Chances are that you can get what you want if you focus your perceptions and cognitions on one thing, in such a way that everything else revolves around it and the rest is ignored.

In the quantum world, reality changes itself according to the observer, and it is hard to say what happens when the observer is absent. We obviously do not live in the quantum world; nevertheless, perception and its illusions can create a unique world for each observer in the scale of the world that we live in.

If you can focus your divine strengths on one goal, the world may change itself for you, and the greatness of your life may surprise you. Do not assume that you know the unknown. The unknown may be scary, because of the stress response and its fear, but it is where all the possibilities live. When you decide to be more than what you are today and to experience, think, and act to make your life as thriving as it can be, you enter into all-new realms of possibility. And this decisive act starts an upward cycle toward strength and joy.

You know a little, and you do not know the limits of human endeavor and sheer will. Do not assume anything, and move toward greatness. Only the future can tell what it holds for you. Your body can even generate new proteins from your inactive genes to deal with the difficulty, and your perception will change as you step into the unknown.

As pointed out earlier, your brain is equipped to turn the potential of the unknown into a predator, but do not get fooled by the folly of your own brain. Move forward and upward.

New experiences in a new world always await you.

The limitation of your mind has its negative side, but the positive side is that you know nothing what you can do, when the potential is endless.

Desires
Motivation is fundamental for life, but it is a double-edged sword. If you are not motivated by a long-term purpose, with a reason, you are likely to be motivated by random, unjustifiable, and transient desires. The motivation to revivify your life with the

truth is good; however, the delusions of desire can let you descend into the darkness.

Goals driven by desires to experience pleasure can be self-destructive and delusory and are often temporary, whereas the purpose that you give to your life does not change easily. Obsessive desires are likely to inflict harm as you deal with complicated matters of life by paralyzing your intellect and fueling irrationality, whereas a purpose has the potential to activate your powerful and positive neural circuits of challenge response.

Finding a meaning for life is difficult intellectual work that takes time and reason, and it involves thinking about the whole, connecting various areas of your brain in a healthy way, whereas a transient desire usually arises from a tiny part of your memory, which wins the war (of neural circuits) to enter into your consciousness.

You may need to read the great philosophical literature or stories to find clues that help you to make sense of everything known and unknown, as it is impossible for just one brain to understand everything. Einstein was able to do what he did in physics because the scientific framework was already in place, and a stable society was established by the sacrifice of countless brave souls.

The stories of humankind and philosophy can give you practical strategies to thrive among the good, bad, and evil of individuals, family, society, and nature, and you are open to use science (applied sciences) as a tool to survive and thrive. Science and art together can help you to find a purpose for life, whereas those who tell you one explanation for everything are wrong and naive.

You need to find a purpose, with scientific and philosophical truth on your side, not arbitrary desires for pleasure arising from the cues in the internal and external worlds. When you live in harmony with the objective and subjective worlds, you become wise and strong; and being naive and weak is generally not good as you deal with the convoluted problems of life.

Pain and Pleasure

We have already discussed that pain and pleasure are not the end goals of life. They just guide you to reach your goal, by providing emotional feedback on the utility and accuracy of your cognitions and actions. Having only pleasure as an end goal can easily reward you with pain, not pleasure.

Even if your end goal is happiness, pursuing a purpose can be the best bet for you because of incentive rewards, which are discussed next.

Rewards

Rewards are of two types: consummatory reward, which you get when you consume a reward—like eating food, and incentive reward, which you get from the hope for a better or exciting future.

Consummatory rewards leave you satiated in the moment as the motivation framework, which motivates you to seek a reward, lives out its purpose. For example, when you are hungry, you seek food, and after eating it, you feel satisfied, and that is it.

There are only a few primary motivators: thirst, hunger, survival, thermoregulation, and reproduction; and primary rewards are generally not enough for lasting happiness for a powerful human brain, which is capable of doing much more. Consummatory rewards of primary motivators are unlikely to keep you happy on a continual basis, because you cannot eat or drink all the time; and habituation, adaptation, and satiation kill the pleasure that you can get from the same consummatory reward.

Incentive rewards, however, can activate dopaminergic pathways for the hope of a better future and employ neural circuits of play and exploration when a difficult purpose is also introduced; and they can completely change the way motivation and emotion influence your life. Hope brings down suffering caused by helplessness or hopelessness, and this hope is not naive optimism. As long as you are alive and have no neurobiological deficiency or disability, your brain can do wonders—but only if you can focus it on a purpose and explore the new or unknown with courage.

The circuits of hope, courage, play, and exploration together can undermine the circuits of fake fear and panic and the rest of the imperfections and illusions; and this is a psychological fact, not an opinion or just optimism.

Hope can be freedom from unrelenting pain (real or illusory), or brand new opportunities, or both. Hope can be for yourself first, and if you can take care of yourself properly, you can extend hope for your family and community, and life itself—which is the purpose of your purpose.

When you have hope for the future, you feel good already because of the incentive reward, and each small success in your pursuit of purpose generates additional positive emotion because of the consummatory reward. Pursuing your purpose is a well-grounded psychological way to experience continual positive emotions, and it can keep negative emotions under control as well.

Hope knows no bounds, because the potential for the collective life is endless, whereas selfish and obsessive desires of consummatory rewards, which concern only the self, often produce misery.

Three States

States of mind and living lifestyles are endless, but in general, there are three ways to live: carrying the pathological baggage of pain (and mental disabilities and disorders); living a usual life with usual stress, boredom, or nihilism; or defining a purpose for your being first, and then charting the course with courage.

Living with unnecessary suffering, which can be avoided or managed with knowledge and skills, is an inferior strategy for living life. Holding on to relentless emotional pain, when it can be controlled, is obviously absurd, and getting rid of neurotic thoughts and behaviors frees you from the tyranny of your own brain.

When you transform yourself (by learning from your past, exploring the new, and becoming wise and strong) your brain can let you leave your painful past behind and make your life normal again. However, normality may not be enough, and with it, the chaotic complexity of life and the weaknesses of the brain can push you back toward the depths of darkness over and over again.

A normal life may not be fulfilling, and chronic stress or boredom or nihilism is often encountered with the normality and sameness. Your brain is negatively biased, and managing stress is a complex cognitive exercise. As pointed out earlier, circuits of courage, play, and exploration can counter a stress response with a challenge response, and there is no other known effective way to manage the stress and the pain, real or illusory. Stress response converts trivial things into metaphorical tigers, and challenge response can bring the unknown potential into your being; and this difference is mind-boggling.

Stress management for just survival becomes easy as you become strong in the pursuit of purpose. Because new information is inevitable as you keep confronting the unknown, boredom is highly unlikely. In general, stress is substituted by boredom, and vice versa, on a regular basis, and a purpose in life can weaken this never-ending cycle of stress and boredom.

Sameness in the form of the known is comforting at times, but it is not sufficient for a flourishing life. The known provides you with a stable platform to stand on, but it is in the wandering into the unknown, searching for the new, where life thrives. A purpose in life changes everything for you, and it is the best strategy to let your life flourish, with new, rich experiences, and with minimal pain, nihilism, stress, and boredom.

Negativity cannot be erased from life; it can be only minimized and managed.

Substance Abuse

Many in the modern world rely on drugs and other substances for happiness; and many substances try to activate the same dopaminergic incentive reward systems artificially that are activated by purpose and its pursuit naturally. This difference is an eye-opener. Drugs unnaturally influence the availability of neurotransmitters in your brain, and any unnatural change in the complicated neurochemistry of the brain by substances causes unintended side effects. Also, the artificial positive emotions wear out soon, leaving you back where you started.

Looking for purpose in your life is the best possible strategy to find authentic happiness (both incentive and consummatory) and live a healthy life without any addictions.

Memory and Meaning

In general, your brain will not let you go away with the painful past, until you make sense of it; and it will not let you live with peace until you find a future purpose.

The primary purpose of your memory is to learn from your positive and negative experiences so that the same mistakes can be avoided and the good experiences can be repeated in the future. Your memory is not just a set of objective facts but also what you have learned according to your subjective experiences with the objective facts—so that you can use it for a better future.

If you make sense of the pain in your past and learn from it and come up with a purpose, your unsettled memories can stop disturbing you; otherwise they will keep disturbing you, and can make you suffer as long as you live. Pain is feedback. Make sense of it, learn from it, come to a philosophical conclusion, and if there is nothing you can do about it, find a purpose and thrive. In this way you can use pain to your advantage.

Transformation

To come up with a purpose for your life, you may also need to find the subjective meaning of the collective life, and that of universe, and beyond. You may need to develop a personal theory of the world, where a lot of visible and invisible things are taken into account.

A sound subjective understanding of the objective world can help you in keeping away the negative emotions that can be activated regularly by an inaccurate map of the world. The unknown is always there, but what is obvious should not be ambiguous for a healthy mind.

Finding a purpose can force you to understand and make sense of the internal and external, the known and unknown. This exercise of transformation needs some serious cognitive efforts and reason, and you emerge wiser and stronger from it, which is in all ways superior to being weak.

If You Do Not Decide Your Purpose, It Will Be Decided for You

Some people just do what they are told, directly or indirectly, and can still live a happy and constructive life. But life is neither simple nor fair. Some win the genetic lottery and others struggle just for health. Some die because they eat too much, whereas others die because there is nothing to eat.

Genes and complex social structures work together to make you the way you are right now, and if you do not like your life right now, then you can make a change by thinking and redefining your philosophy, giving meaning to your life the way you like it, and taking action.

If you do not decide on a direction for your life by yourself, it will be done for you, and you may end up having goals that are good for neither you nor others.

Facts and their interpretations are infinite, and most of them are irrelevant for your survival. Out of the infinite information available, you need finite biological reality (in the form of a subjective purpose or meaning), which can be used as a tool for you to survive and thrive.

This strategy may not be perfect, but it works for all practical purposes, and you cannot wait until all the facts are in. And no one knows if that is ever going to happen. Even if you can know everything, you can focus only on a finite amount at one time, and you can only do finite things in your life.

The meaning of life may be personal for you, but it is in your own interest that it is aligned with the psychological and neurological facts. No one wants to live with misery, but chasing something that leads to misery contradicts your fundamental preferences.

Taking action with a purpose or meaning means moving beyond just survival (or just pain and pleasure) to something great and transcendent, which is hard to understand with a conscious thought. Consciousness is mysterious, and subliminal neural activity deals with the matters that you cannot comprehend consciously, and as you take action to pursue your purpose, subconsciousness will reward you with positive emotions involuntarily.

Deciding on a purpose for your life is the single most important decision that you can make in your life.

TAKE ACTION, BUT NOT FOR REWARDS

You need to take action for your survival but, contrary to other life forms, your life can be more than just survival. You can flourish, too, if you can effectively use your executive cognitive functions. However, thinking about rewards all the time can bring down the efficiency and lucidity of your brain and can even make your survival difficult.

The human brain works in mysterious and silent ways. The physical and psychological actions comprising your life appear to be affected by similar states of mind, but in reality, different mechanism drive efficiency of each kind of action. It turns out that thinking obsessively about rewards improves performance for physical action, but such an infatuation with rewards silently deteriorates cognitive competence and coherence for complex cognitive tasks.

Mechanical and cognitive skills make up a spectrum of skills that help you to chart a course of action amid order and chaos. Mechanical skills require physical resources and efforts, whereas cognitive skills need cognitive counterparts.

As long as the task at hand involves only mechanical skills such as running, thinking about rewards leads to a better performance, and as reward becomes more and more valuable, execution of physical action becomes increasingly efficient.

When the task at hand requires a cognitive skill rather than a physical one—complex problem-solving, for example—obsessive thinking about prizes could potentially lead to poorer cognitive performance; and as the obsession for rewards intensifies, the quality of cognitive action can become progressively worse.

Neither success nor happiness in the modern world can be achieved by physical action only. You must take cognitive action, but the efficiency of it could be compromised by an excessive expectation of reward.

Thinking about rewards brings down your cognitive performance by interfering with other cognitive processes in several ways.

Wanting a reward, and actual cognitive processes which try to translate your imagined reward into reality, need some same shared cognitive resources (short-term memory and focus for example) to run; and the more you think about rewards, the fewer cognitive resources will be allocated to actual problem-solving processes.

In the worst case, compulsive thinking about rewards can completely occupy your cognitive resources, leaving no room for productive problem-solving processes to run at all.

Another major problem with the rewards being the focal point of your thoughts is that switching your focus from one cognitive process to another is effortful and difficult. Thoughts of rewards, or fear of not getting the reward, could go on and on for a long time before you can cognitively switch your focus back to actually productive work.

Thinking about what you want or do not want is not enough in itself, and as thoughts of reward come back to mind again and again, switching back to actual beneficial work becomes increasingly difficult.

Similarly to having multiple cognitions (thoughts or cognitive processes) in your consciousness, a personal computer runs software (also called apps, applications, or processes) with the help of the computational resources of the central processing unit (CPU) and short-term memory (RAM), among others.

However, each software program is run for a fraction of a second in the CPU, and then another program is run from the list of all currently running programs by performing a context switch. A context switch stops one program, saves its current data and state, loads data and the state of the next program in the queue, and runs it. This happens very quickly, many times in a second, as though all the open apps were running in parallel. However, in general, only one program can run at a time. And when a program cannot be stopped from running, other software cannot run, and your computer or mobile device gets hung up. You can either kill the process with the process manager or restart your device.

Also, a context switch in the computer is expensive computationally, but a cognitive switch is much more difficult for the human brain—and sometimes impossible.

A computer, however, has a restart button that can erase all apps from the short-term memory and start fresh, whereas we do not have such a cognitive reset.

Your brain may resemble a computer in computing information, but it is not the same as a computer. The brain has an intelligent motivation framework, which computers do not have as of today. However, freezing in a computer or mobile phone is an excellent real-life example of how an obsessive cognition or emotion or desire or belief can corrupt your consciousness.

A desire, or the focus on its reward, is not enough to consume the wanted reward. In many cases, you must take other cognitive actions, and keep learning from the painful feedbacks, maybe for years, before you can enjoy the rewards. And an obsessive focus on rewards only cannot let other cognitive processes run that can help you get what you want.

Focusing obsessively on rewards is wasting your most important cognitive currency—focus, which can direct other cognitive resources for your benefit. Prosperity in life is easier when you actively use your faculty of cognition; however, it is of no use when it is drawn primarily toward rewarding thoughts only.

Taking action for rewards may fuel fear of failure. When stakes are extremely high and cognitive action is needed, fear will initiate a stress response that is designed to hijack your rational brain.

Fear is good for physical action because a stress response helps your body perform better physically, but fear is toxic for your cognitive abilities. During critical moments (for example: an exam for which you have been preparing for years, approaching a potential romantic partner, or attending a job interview or business meeting), fear can introduce complete cognitive paralysis.

Low-resolution survival software can also freeze you mentally and physically when you are faced with real or illusory fearful emotions. Most fear or panic in the modern world is fake, and when you do not care about the result of each action, you are saved from most of it—and from the probable cognitive paralysis associated with it.

It has been discussed before that a prediction of pleasure that you expect to receive from a reward in the future could be delusional, due to the limits of your brain and a range of cognitive illusions; and excessive focus on reward facilitates even more compelling and powerful illusions. Delusional obsession on reward further reduces your cognitive efficiency, and actually does the opposite of what it pretends to achieve.

Along with hedonic prediction, you cannot predict objective outcome of your actions accurately all the time. Under uncertainty, a wrong prediction will make you quit, even when there is a huge probability of success in the near future. If you are dealing with the important matters of life and randomness at the same time, taking action anyway regardless of its outcome is a superior strategy to giving up.

Not doing anything ensures complete failure, whereas relentless action often opens doors to success. Luck plays an important role in any huge success and may turn in your favor if there is enough effort. You can never know how close to success you are in any complicated domain. You may need to work on many things at many levels. Even when success is close, it may appear too far, and vice versa. In such situations, continuing to take action regardless of positive or negative rewards can help you succeed sooner or later.

Life and the world are more complex than they appear to be, and things are connected and controlled in known and unknown ways. You can control or predict result of a rudimentary task, but you cannot do the same for complex ventures. Years of physical and cognitive action may not be enough for some goals, and when execution is often greeted with failures, reward-seeking behavior will slow you down.

If reward is what you want from each action, then doing what you do not like could be miserable, and you may opt out of your responsibilities. You may not like all the courses in school, or you may not like your job, but you cannot always run away from something that is not enjoyable, and if you do, opportunities can be missed and problems may arise.

Modern-day problems that we face at school, business, work, and home cannot be solved by physical skills alone. More importantly we need cognitive skills; and learning to take action without compulsive wanting of rewards retains our cognitive clarity and our ability to use cognitive skills in an efficient manner.

Whenever you learn something new, your brain strengthens connections among corresponding neurons, and it takes time, efforts, pain, and repetition. The neuroplasticity of your brain can even create new neural circuits for a new skill and rewire old circuits used for a different skill. The key is recurring and consistent cognitive action.

Bracing yourself for regular failures encountered during mental exertions and not getting swayed by them requires that you keep on going regardless of the positive or negative outcome. Building psychological strengths with massive cognitive action is not necessarily pleasant, but not wanting rewards for each and every action can make your journey even joyful.

You can focus only finite at a time. Hence, the action-focused mindset, which does not care about results all of the time, makes you cognitively efficient by helping you live in the present (once a purpose is found and a plan is prepared) and focus on the task at hand, for the better execution.

A purpose must be accompanied by a plan, and a long-term plan must be divided into short-term tasks (maybe hourly), and the successful and efficient execution of each of these tasks is the key to success. Learning can be analyzed periodically, but focusing on the small task at hand, not on its reward, is critical for the execution.

You may want the reward of each of your actions, but it is not in your direct control always. You can imagine an exciting and glittering future, and take action as you try to approach the final reward; however, gratification from the consumption of the reward is not always possible, and potential failure is not comforting.

You can think about finding a job or a date, or starting a business, and you can certainly act, but you can never control the result of each of your actions. And when your wishes wither away without being materialized, which usually happens too often, dejection can create much more pain than the habituating happiness which can be generated by the rewards.

Simple rewards can be enjoyed by anyone, but the end result of a series of complex and prolonged tasks cannot be controlled by you single-handedly. An employee may fantasize about becoming CEO one day, but no one can enforce it, no matter how much talent and expertise that one has. An entrepreneur cannot enforce success if operating in a complex territory, and you cannot always marry the love of your life, and the list goes on and on.

Huge success hangs on unlimited strands of a complex whole, accompanied by an almost perfect amalgamation of nature and nurture, luck and talent, industry and courage; and still you cannot run away from action, even if the result is not in your control always.

The world is not fair, and expecting rewards for each and every action can turn into a wretched nightmare easily, when you are dealing with convoluted ongoing matters of life. Not focusing on the rewards, and moving from one action to another, saves you from much of the misery that you may go through in the completion of a complex task.

Not only what you think about outcome of your actions but

judgement of others, when they are evaluating your actions, can also lead to decline in your creative problem solving. Not caring about the result of each and every one of your actions saves you from yourself, and from others as well.

Taking action without expecting anything in return, increases your probability of success. When dealing with randomness and complexity, you cannot guarantee success, and increasing your chances of success is all that you can do.

TAKE ACTION, EVEN IF IT IS IMPERFECT

Defects in your actions are inevitable, and you should not stop taking action because of that.

The human brain is finite, and it struggles to manage the infinite. In general, a new endeavor is going to be full of imperfections, learning, and pain. Cognitive and physical action must not be stopped, even if imperfection is embedded in it. Your perception and internal representations of the external world will always be limited, and you can never prepare yourself perfectly for the new or infinite.

The world has a static and dynamic nature, and what you do today with a great degree of accuracy may not be enough in the future; what works today may seem flawed tomorrow. Out of infinite possibilities, you cannot learn every skill needed for every possibility, and your errors guide you to correct your thinking and behavior for the task at hand.

You obviously cannot avoid mistakes, but same mistakes should not be repeated over and over again when there is no need for it. We have discussed that while trying to learn a new explicit skill (driving a car, for example), the same errors must be repeated over a few weeks, and as the frequency of your errors increases, you learn faster.

Contrary to conventional wisdom, errors are often your friends. Sometimes you cannot avoid making mistakes, but you get useful feedback from the errors, and at other times the unambiguous feedback of your repeated errors makes you learn a new skill. Errors are inevitable in survival, and a life that tries to flourish is subjected to even more errors of a different kind.

The limits of the human brain ensure that your knowledge is always limited, and when you work on new challenges, most of your actions are subject to error. You cannot know everything in advance, and when you step voluntarily into the unknown, where all the possibilities reside, novel errors are your constant companions.

The path to creativity and growth cannot be perfectly defined in advance, and the imperfections of your actions push you toward your subjective perfection. Taking action, knowing that it is likely to have defects, you do not fear failure, and by doing so you expose yourself to boundless possibilities without being paralyzed by perfectionism.

Defects in your actions may not be comfortable, but it is through them that your life can be made to blossom.

It may be obvious that a thriving and exciting life is generally not possible without physical and psychological action; however, people primarily prefer not to move from their couch or flex a cognitive muscle. Our minds and bodies long for lousy laziness, but life cannot exist without physical action, and adequate satisfaction in life is unlikely to be found in the absence of constructive cognitive action.

Erasing indolence one takes action, although taxing exertions can cause stress, and not taking enough demanding actions may bring boring discomfort. Furthermore, without the motivation of rewards, action seems meaningless, and yet compulsive desire for consummatory rewards breeds cognitively inefficiency and misery.

One may want a positive outcome of every action, but one can never control the result of each action, and one cannot not take action, and not liking day-to-day activities makes life ineffectual and miserable.

The brain is all-powerful and mysterious and has spectacular subliminal strengths that are beyond our conscious comprehension; and its weaknesses make us suffer.

Several neural circuits of the brain seduce us in a multitude of directions in an incoherent manner; and the authenticity of each path is not clear. Internal chaos or infinite cosmos, wonders of the brain, can easily be converted into weaknesses without long-term leadership.

The motivation framework is formidable, and each of its elements makes us suffer with laziness, inaction, or arbitrary action. Action is absolutely necessary for survival, but the brain does not let us live in peace even when survival is taken care of.

The path of action is puzzling, and the solution lies in meaningful action in which one transcends beyond hedonic motivation to find a higher meaning in life and, without begging for gratification from each action, engages in activities that give life a moral significance and direction, despite the defects in one's actions.

One can transcend beyond survival and decide on a subjective reason to exist, explore, and act; and as meaningful action is taken, continual positive emotions are generated genuinely, without any obsessive expectation of pleasure from the consumption of rewards. And, no, science can never define the meaning of your life or that of collective life. At least not today.

Science is a list of abstractions, and origins of abstractions are still mysterious. An abstraction defines what is, and creates a range of possibilities for you with in its laws. However, scientific abstractions cannot define a subjective possibility for you, and you are always free to decide what you should be in your life.

The meaning of your life is the continual leadership, giving you courage and confidence to confront chaos and complexity, known and unknown, head-on. Taking meaningful action is one of the needs of your brain, and without it you suffer, and your existence withers away.

FOCUS AND MEDITATION

Focus is the forefront of your cognitive faculties and it can direct all other neural resources and processes, one way or another.

Meditation is learning to control your attention by attempting to deliberately direct it on any one particular thing (for example: your breath, the tip of your nose, a word, a mantra, silence, or any other finite thing) for a period of time. Meditation is often encountered in yoga, where the focus is primarily on a word (om, for example), but you can focus on anything that is fixed. Meditation is a form of cognitive yoga (cognitive exercise), and other popular forms of yoga are breathing and stretching exercises.

Your mind wanders as you struggle to focus, but you aim your attention back to your focal point over and over again. What looks like a simple act of fixating your consciousness on one thing may be incredibly challenging at first, but just a few months of daily practice alters your brain and behavior in remarkably positive ways. A few are discussed in this chapter.

The amygdala is a region in your brain associated with heightened levels of stress and anxiety, and meditation triggers a decrease in its volume. An overacting amygdala wreaks havoc in life, but the meditation causes its shrinkage and in turn increases its utility.

Meditation has also been correlated with a fitter and more youthful cortex, which is the part of the brain responsible for executing higher cognitive functions. The hippocampus in your brain is associated with learning and memory, and meditation increases its gray-matter volume.

Meditation also leads to increased activity in the left prefrontal cortex, which is linked to emotions of joy. Meditation helps in the maintenance of your genes by protecting the length of the protective caps at the end of chromosomes called telomeres, which erode with age.

Meditation promotes neural plasticity, aids longevity and learning, preserves cognition, and increases blood flow in certain regions of the brain.

A daily practice of mediation helps in enhancing perceptual receptivity, discrimination, and openness, and leads to decreased cognitive reaction times, improved cognitive efficiency and flexibility, superior memory, less habituation, and better problem-solving.

The efforts of abstinence from mental or physical movement during meditation provide a therapeutic delay and enable you to judge your thoughts and behaviors before reacting. This sense of self-control blunts destructive compulsions and urges, boosting self-esteem in the process. We have already discussed the absolute need for self-control in life, and meditation is one of the ways to develop it.

Meditation triggers a relaxation response with a series of healthy physiological changes: slow heartbeat and respiration, lower blood pressure, and reduced lactate levels in the blood. As pointed out earlier, the relaxation response is the opposite of the fight-or-flight stress response, and when it is initiated, harmful physiological and psychological changes associated with the stress response come to an abrupt temporary end.

In addition to cognitive stress, the relaxation response also helps guard against oxidative stress—the bodily damage caused by free radicals. The relaxation response is one of the primary strategies for managing the ongoing stress of life (along with the challenge response), and meditation is a simple way to activate it.

Meditation is likely to help if you are dealing with depression, anxiety, stress disorders, aggression, addiction, chronic pain and medical illnesses, insomnia, and hypertension, and it is highly likely to be suggested during cognitive behavioral therapy (CBT).

Attending to a focal point and keeping the mind from wandering acts as a catalyst in the growth of self-awareness, self-control, sustained focus, detachment, and cognitive switching (switching from one cognitive process to another). This set of cognitive competencies acquired during meditation powers your powerful cognitive machinery to focus on what matters most for you in the infinite cosmos.

Taking control of your focus is not possible without self-awareness, and awareness of your thoughts and behaviors may be problematic in the short run as you realize the folly of your own brain and beliefs, but it is pragmatic in the long run.

Awareness of the contents of your consciousness may guide you to see things differently than before and may let your left and right cerebral hemispheres communicate in new ways, creating possibilities for a new type of thinking where a complex whole makes some sense, and complex problems can be solved.

Once you learn to control your attention, your brain can generalize it, and you can direct it to anything you wish at your will. For example, focusing on your major muscles one by one and releasing all the unwanted muscle tension triggers a relaxation response, which is one of the easiest way to reverse harmful changes initiated by the stress response.

In being equanimous, instead of your breath or a word, you focus on your cognitions and emotions with an indifferent, unafraid, and detached state of mind, and as a result, your consciousness can be prevented from corruption by its own contents.

You can focus on action, which gives a purpose or meaning to your life, without expecting rewards from each action, and such focus starts an upward journey toward excellence. Focusing on action, to manifest your destiny in reality and just because you can—such a shift in focus can make all the difference in your life.

The list goes on.

Cognitive processes or neural circuits, no matter how intellectual or powerful they may be, are of no use if they cannot be retrieved from your long-term memory, held in your consciousness, and acted upon. You are much more powerful than you think you are, in spite of all of the cruelty and complexity of life.

However, super-heroic strengths in you can do nothing if you cannot use your focus to aim them at something meaningful, and you are frequently distracted by worthless things instead.

No one knows what you can do, receive, and give until you commit to a purpose for your existence, stop or override all other cognitive or emotional noise in your head, learn to aim all that you have got at one thing, do not beg for rewards from each of your action, and take massive action (cognitive and physical) with a final resolve, even if the action has imperfections embedded in it.

ACQUIRE KNOWLEDGE

Darkness dwells in this world, and in your head; it is knowledge which lights up the darkness.

Living in the prison of pathological pain or being philosophically stagnant in the flow of time are not the optimal use of the divine powers vested in you. Suffering or stress are not the only forces in this world, and one can reverse the course, upward toward blossom, with knowledge.

The information that you hold in your memory is never enough and not always accurate, because your memory is bounded by the number of neurons in your head, and your nervous system is not perfect. From time to time, objective facts are required to make an addition in your memory and corrections in your cognitions.

Your cognitions and emotions seem to be sourced from the deep layers of subconsciousness, and the accuracy or relevance of those is complicated by several primal and novel neural systems working together in an incoherent way. You cannot always believe in your thoughts and emotions blindly, and the significance of this fact cannot be overstated.

Information in this world is infinite. Your assumptions about what you know and do not know and the validity of your assumptions, together, fabricate your personal reality. Sometimes what you know is not real, and sometimes what is real you do not know. The cocktail of known and unknown, real and unreal is confusing.

Reality here means everything that can let you survive and thrive with least amount of suffering—and with knowledge you can at least erase ambiguity, when it is certainly possible to do so.

Knowledge protects you from the unnecessary suffering inflicted by internal irrationality and provides strategies to alleviate pain, and a use the unavoidable pain for your benefit. And most importantly, keeping the weaknesses of your brain under control, knowledge can awaken its sleeping strengths, which can let you prosper.

The stunning complexity of the world is ever present. You may have been protected from it so far, but it can reveal itself in a flick of a switch. A betrayal, a rejection, a tragedy, a survival struggle, a dream crushed, and the like all can cause you to question your limited internal abstraction of the external world, but knowledge can prevent your downfall, especially when life strikes on multiple fronts.

How knowledge can affect your hedonic motivation, health, and success is discussed next.

KNOWLEDGE AND THE HEDONIC MOTIVATION

Knowledge can discriminate between good and bad; without it, self-destructive or useless behavior may seem rewarding or essential. A course of action cannot be corrected in the absence of awareness of its flaws, and knowledge is the first line of defense against deeply ingrained irrational behavior.

For example, an optical illusion appears real if you do not know about it already. In the same manner, if you do not know about cognitive illusions in advance, absurd cognitions (and emotions) may seem authentic, without a shadow of doubt. Illusions of thought (and emotion) can make you suffer more than that is unavoidable, and awareness of the illusions is the first step to stop or supersede the unnecessary suffering.

The hedonic principle prevails over human existence in a self-defeating manner, and in the absence of knowledge of such self-inflicted wounds, one lives in the superfluous horrors of self-deception. Knowledge diminishes the darkness of imperfect and incompetent intelligence by exposing the facade of predictable and personal pitfalls disguised as rationality.

Life is generally good only if exaggerations of experiences of pain and pleasure do not interfere in your daily struggle, and such exaggerations are common for materialistic and other endless possibilities of the modern world.

A life where fundamental needs (access to food, family, and social security) are fulfilled is a pretty good life, but modern life may corrupt your mind with imagined pleasures from the endless supply of materialistic things. But, truth be told, such imagination is just an illusion in the long run. There is nothing wrong in pursuing materialistic things, but it is when greed takes away your ability to think clearly and peace that you may be in trouble.

Desiring luxury may be okay when your desire does not rob you of your executive functions and clarity of mind; but if you cannot find peace in the presence of the most critical things, useless or luxurious things cannot guarantee long-term satisfaction either.

Cognitive illusions coupled with wanting could amplify the imagined exaggerations of pleasures to insanity, and in case your desires are fulfilled, habituation will soon convert the new to nothing. With knowledge of habituation (and adaptation and satiation), you can reach a logical conclusion that luxuries or other psychological objects are nice to have, but they cannot make your life fulfilling forever.

Materialistic things can give your happiness a temporary boost on occasion, but in the course of time, you will get back to your usual state of mind. Money and materialistic things are not a complete solution to the complex problems of life, and this knowledge suggests you to develop alternative cognitive skills and find a purpose that can handle the life the way it is.

In general, your states of mind are regulated by your focus, and your ability to control your focus and keep it on positive emotions—by conscious efforts or by finding and pursuing a purpose—matters much more than materialism and money.

With knowledge you know that pain and pleasure are emotional guides, not the end goals; and an obsessive pursuit of pleasure (with pain intolerance) can easily become the paradoxical pursuit of pain, not pleasure.

Learning to acknowledge and appreciate the good already in life, and going after what is meaningful, are some of the most reliable ways to bring positive emotions into being, whereas chasing a mirage in the hope of eternal happiness will keep disappointment alive.

It is already tragic that there is so much real suffering in this world, but to suffer without any actual misfortune because of an illusory hunger for things is a downright disgrace to human intelligence. Knowledge of illusions can regulate or reverse the cognitive or emotional noise in your head, and as a result you can use your cognitive resources to face the real and unavoidable challenges of life.

Illusions appear real, and without a careful and critical evaluation of your thoughts, you are likely to believe them as they arise, no matter how unjustifiable they may be. Knowledge can, however, reveal the façade of unreal reality.

When you know how cognitions and emotions can automatically arise in the head, and how the dualities of desire and disgust can delude you toward self-destruction, you react to your cognitions and emotions with reason (on the basis of factual knowledge), not just because they pop up in your head.

In the wild, survival is the only need of life, and before the scientific revolution, cravings were still extremely limited for most, but now desires know no bounds. Science has helped humanity in numerous ways, but it has also created the widespread destruction of nature, when it became entangled with the very thing that made its development possible—human brain.

Desire for instant gratification and never ending greed, together, have started a race that is self-defeating both for people and for the planet. The information that you get from corporate advertisements, formal education, mainstream media, political propaganda, and other common sources is unlikely to be for your welfare—or that of Mother Earth, for that matter.

You need knowledge to stop the use and abuse of your life by those who try to manipulate your psychological vulnerabilities. The management of pain and pleasure is marinated in complexity and uncertainty, and if pain is in abundance in your life, knowledge can make all the difference.

KNOWLEDGE AND HEALTH

Your physical and psychological health depends on several factors, and access to medical care is usually not unlimited. Physical and mental health professionals can obviously help, but it is your knowledge about cognitive and physical fitness that matters most.

We have discussed a lot about the psychological aspects of cognitive fitness; however, purely biological aspects can also make a difference.

An imbalance of just one vitamin, mineral, neurotransmitter, or hormone can change how you feel, and a simple test can provide information that can save you from your misery. For example, too much thyroid hormone can trigger maniac episodes, and depression can be because of too little thyroid hormone. In many cases, a hormone supplement may be all that is needed to feel normal again.

Lower levels of the neurotransmitter serotonin can cause depression as well, and a SSRI (selective serotonin reuptake inhibitor) can help in a month. Similarly, a vitamin B12 deficiency, especially in vegetarians and old people, can cause depressive symptoms.

Your energy levels also affect how you feel, and energy generation is dependent on many chemicals and your circadian rhythm. Going to bed and waking up at the same time can help in mood disorders. Eating a healthy and balanced breakfast is usually good for your energy levels and cognitive function.

Your mood depends on a lot of chemicals and several systems, and knowledge of the imbalance of chemicals or a problem with any system is not always obvious. If your moods are not in your control most of the time, a simple test can provide a single piece of information that you may need to normalize your moods again. Otherwise, a personality transformation can always assist.

Not only psychological distress but the chances of developing several chronic diseases can be cut down with the latest scientific knowledge. Having information that can prevent mental and physical disease and disability is extremely crucial, because every condition is not curable.

A balanced diet of fresh fruits and vegetables, whole grains, complex carbohydrates, lean protein, and good fats (high monounsaturated fat, polyunsaturated fat, and fish oil; minimum saturated fat and almost no trans fat), along with muscular, cardiovascular, cognitive, breathing (yoga), and stretching exercises will improve your physical and psychological health and posture, whereas a mentally and physically sedentary lifestyle combined with poor eating habits can cost you dearly.

Exposure to harmful pollutants and radiation or an imbalance of vitamins, minerals, fat, proteins, carbohydrates, neurotransmitters, hormones, and the rest contribute to a number of miserable medical conditions, which can be cured, prevented, or managed with knowledge, within the bounds of possibility.

For example, carcinogens can give you cancer; trans fats, simple carbohydrates, and bad cholesterol are likely to introduce chronic medical conditions; and the list goes on and on. Prevention is critical, as cure is not always feasible.

Also, you can delay the downfall of general intelligence (IQ) as you age with anaerobic and aerobic physical exercise.

Knowledge of how physical posture can affect your mood and mobility also matters. Bad physical posture can lead to skeletal deformity and loss of function, and good physical posture improves your appearance and facilitates a positive and confident mood.

Knowledge of good and bad ways to stand or sit (for example, stand or sit straight, with shoulders back and abdomen tucked in), and awareness of muscular and stretching exercises, which help you to maintain a good physical posture, can prevent future disability, deformity, and negative moods.

Body and mind can prime each other in mysterious ways, and a good mental and physical posture can be your conscious choice. By default, negativity may crowd our consciousness, and slouching is common in the world of computers and mobile phones.

Self-control can keep track of your cognitive and physical postures and makes changes on demand.

A few critical things are summarized in this book for your good health, and there is a lot to know. The aim here is to outline the absolute importance of knowledge for your overall fitness and well-being. Medical science is updated on a daily basis, and it is in your interest to be aware of the critical updates.

Knowledge is important for your health, but without having broad knowledge of how to take control back from an irrational and primitive brain, a single piece of accurate information could also be useless. For example, just knowing smoking can cause cancer is usually never enough to quit.

We have discussed how advanced knowledge of the life cycle of desire and disgust can prevent the substance dependence from arising in the first place, and such knowledge can free you from an existing substance subjugation.

KNOWLEDGE AND SUCCESS

Learning is acquiring new knowledge or skills from experiences, which can change the thought and behavior of the learner; however, learning usually takes time, effort, and blunders. Life is too short to learn everything on your own, and the available collective wisdom can save you from wasting your precious limited time.

Mistakes and blunders are inevitable and intermittent as you advance toward your purpose, and not all but many of them may be avoided by knowledge. With factual knowledge, success can be an easy routine in some areas, like passing an exam or being efficient in usual jobs. And if you are dealing with complexity and uncertainty, in your job or in your venture, the probability of success can rise with knowledge.

An illusion of learning manifests when you just read and do not test yourself occasionally. An illusion will not help you in passing a difficult exam. Limited information available in the short-term memory gives rise to an illusion of detailed information stored in the long-term memory, and a test can reveal what is actually learned (encoded and stored in the memory for the future retrieval).

Knowledge can provide clues for success in all areas of life—

not only in schools and colleges. For success, technical skills alone may not be enough, and you may need cognitive skills, which allocate your cognitive resources accordingly, especially when the going gets tough, and your mind is distracted by frequent feedback of failures and negative emotions.

Cognitive resilience, which can prevent your cognitive clarity from degrading into confusion and paralysis, may matter more than your technical skills in many cases. However, cognitive skills that you need for a goal are not obvious always, and knowledge can help you in the discovery and development of psychological strengths, without which success is sometimes just not possible.

You are likely to be rejected as many as forty-nine times to get a job interview or to find a date, and in general, the rate of success in most of the critical and difficult things is just around 2 percent. You are likely to fail most of the time, and you only need to be right just once. With the knowledge of this fact and equanimity with courage, you can keep learning from your failures and ultimately succeed.

Knowledge also helps you to make empowering associations, rather than correlating things completely out of proportion. When you realize that the brain is inherently irrational and heuristic, you do not label irrational behavior as a personal flaw. Personal beliefs or cognitive illusions that do not help need to be changed or managed, and realizing how they got into your head in the first place takes the burden or guilt off your shoulders.

Using self-compassion (as you change your thought and behavior for good) and knowing that you did not choose your genes or childhood habitat, you do not beat yourself up for your objective or subjective imperfections. It does not mean that you do not take responsibility for your thought and behavior, but it is about being realistic about how nervous system can be changed.

Change becomes easier with knowledge of the psychological forces that give rise to thought and behavior and keep them alive. Knowing that no one is perfect, and that blunders are part of the process, you keep learning; but do not beat yourself up for the inevitable, and do not stop.

Happiness or prosperity are generally not the default choices for most, but out of infinite directions, you can always define a definitive moral transcendent direction for your life. Your brain can never manage infinity, but it can sure chase a specific goal and generate positive emotions along the way, despite difficulties and complexities on the long-term path that you decide to tread.

There are a number of systems and roles in your head, and each can be compared to a separate entity and personality. If you do not define which identity has a final say, you are subjected to internal chaos, too, in addition to the external. There are an infinite number of things to do in an infinite number of ways in this universe, and knowledge can suggest what is important for you.

Without knowledge, you may live a life devoid of any purpose or meaning, and complexity may rule and eventually ruin your life, producing pain even in the most serene and beautiful moments. Knowledge and strategies introduced in this book assist you to think critically and solve complex problems as you try to attain your subjectively meaningful goals, which define your success.

Obsessive desires or unrelenting negative emotions are usually not favorable for your success, and a few fundamental strategies are proposed in this book so that you can deal with the hostility of your own brain. Along with positive and courageous states of mind, your performance for success also depends on your energy levels and overall health. If your energy levels are low, consultation with a doctor to check any imbalance of chemicals (hormones, neurotransmitters, vitamins, and minerals, among others) can change your life. Your lifestyle or eating habits also affect your energy levels. For example, a lack of water, iron, magnesium, vitamin B12, sleep, breakfast, or exercise or excess of sugar, alcohol, or stress can lower your energy levels.

Cognitive fitness helps you to regulate your sleep, stress and, alcohol intake, and a doctor can check and provide supplements for any biological deficiency.

It is always hard to believe, but sometimes just one chemical can make you suffer for your whole life, and this is one of the reason why the knowledge of complexity can absolutely matter.

A modern-day sedentary lifestyle can ruin your physical health and posture, and acquisitiveness or decadence can make you suffer even in the absence of any real struggle. Modern life presents physical and cognitive challenges that were absent in the old days, and to safely navigate through the new world of information overload, you need knowledge.

You can control your physical, psychological, and existential destiny with advanced knowledge of internal and external worlds, whereas general knowledge is generally a product of groupthink or the collective irrationality of humanity, and it can produce predictably miserable results.

Pleasure and pain are not the opposite ends of single continuum. We have discussed that pain is obviously unwanted, but the absence of pain does not guarantee pleasure, and management of pain and pleasure is neither obvious nor simple.

The human brain and the world—both are complicated. If you have knowledge of the objective and subjective worlds (including the social world) and how they interact with each other, you can correct your thoughts and beliefs accordingly so that you do not fight an already lost battle.

Arrogance or ignorance may work, at least for you, when your survival, emotional support, social security, and health are protected by your environment and genes, but not all are born in privileged families with near-perfect active genes.

Dissatisfaction in life when fundamental needs are fulfilled is easier to erase with knowledge. And if resources are rare in your life and uncertainties are in abundance, making your survival difficult or miserable, then—with the help of knowledge—you can still minimize the chaos and complexities in your life. However, it may not be easy at first.

In this book, we have presented a few facts and strategies for you to think clearly. It is up to you to think, gain knowledge, experience the new, and solve the problems of your life; and cognitive fitness is the lifelong hunger for new experiences, wisdom, and strength in the uncertain and changing world.

You live in a socioeconomic world with a biological body, among other known and unknown things, and a problem in your life can be because of multiple factors in multiple domains, many of which may or may not be in your direct or indirect control. A suggestion that one idea can work in every situation is absurd, and nothing could be further from the truth. Cognitive fitness may appear as one idea but it is experiencing new, gaining knowledge and becoming strong in the numerous layers of several roles and domains.

Knowledge works with the available objective information, and your subjective imagination to make sense of your past, current, and future place in the eternal cosmos; and it can also suggest strategies to minimize and manage the suffering of life. Without knowledge health, happiness, and prosperity are generally a product of randomness, and it does not favor everyone.

Life is already difficult, and being intellectually blind generally makes it worse.

CONCLUSION

Success is subjective.

Huge success is fascinating, and many people who have tasted it rely on drugs, alcohol, and other substances for happiness. The drug industry has become the major industry trying to sell happiness, alongside of consumerism, but after the initial euphoria, the mind adapts to it, and many die from drug overdoses—including some well-known, super successful celebrities.

Clearly there is something missing in the stories of success when you take an outward look at them. Writers of those stories can neither recreate the past to know exactly how success unfolded nor predict the future with certainty to forecast the effects of success on the well-being of a person.

Instead of admitting their ignorance, they give you their subjective and delusional version of the story, but it is only a tiny part of the whole, infected by focusing illusion and overconfidence.

The definition of success may be different for each of us, but an essential and first part of any success is the ability to appreciate the presence of positives (and the absence of negatives) in life, as well as the strength to exert authority over irrational cognitions and emotions in the head.

Once you are able to do that, you like your life already in most cases, and one can argue that this is the real success.

Furthermore, the probability of your success in the future rises with the enhanced cognitive efficiency of a grateful positive state of mind; and if you are victorious, your victory could stay that way.

If you cannot feel gratitude for the indispensable things (habitable environment, your existence, health, social security, and love, to name a few), you are not likely to find any long-term happiness from other things, either. Your brain habituates to things which are most important than anything else, and other emotions or man-made materialistic things stand no chance against brutal habituation, adaptation, and satiation.

The wisest people ever to walk on this planet lived the simplest lives, where there was a lack of things but an abundance of wisdom, and struggling to find enough exhilaration in the abundance of things is a well-established trend of the modern world.

Suffering does exist in existence, and external factors playing their part in the presence of pain is plain to see for all. However, most of the misery lurking in your life does not come from the outside; it is manufactured right inside your head.

Whatever the case may be, the faculty of rational or intelligent thought, acquiring knowledge of higher order, experiencing and exploring the unknown for new information and potential, and developing fundamental cognitive strengths are always a part of the solution. And this is what cognitive fitness aims to achieve.

Cognitive fitness is the underlying leadership that holds perceptions, thoughts, emotions, actions, motivations, imagination, and illusory intelligence together in such a way that suffering is minimal and happiness is possible.

Cognitive stimulation, stress management, eating a healthy, plant-based diet, getting enough sleep, building social connections, and physical exercise are some primary strategies usually suggested for cognitive fitness. These strategies help; however, psychological fitness is much more convoluted and puzzling than is presumed.

The cognitive illusions, hidden habits, blind beliefs, and invisible ingrained tricks and functions of your brain are endless, and even one can be enough to take away your clarity of mind and peace, even without any genuine problems in your life.

Suffering is an unavoidable part of your being, and ironically, the absence of any authentic suffering is not necessarily an improvement in your experience of happiness.

Acting as an adversary, your mind may not help you in your struggle by itself if you do not know how to control it. You can analyze your cognitions and actions (and resulting emotions) over a period of time, but you cannot manage all of them instantly, in each moment, for consistent rational cognitive action that solves the problems of life without creating new ones, and for this reason you need a few fundamental cognitive strategies that somehow can win the war against the self-betrayal of your own brain and the chaos of the external world.

Knowledge of the complexity of internal and external worlds and illusions; facing the dualities of life with courage and equanimity; exercising self-control over cognitions, emotions, actions, and attention; making sense of the internal and external world, and aiming your neural machinery toward a meaningful goal; and taking action for the purpose of your being, not rewards are some of the fundamental strategies that, when practiced enough, become exceptional psychological assets.

Cognitive fitness is the force that weakens the weaknesses of your brain and awakens your intellect, strength, and courage to win the battle against internal and external chaos and complexities. This war is fought at various fronts and lasts for lifetime, so that you do not lose yourself in a labyrinth of complexity.

Pain and pleasure are unavoidable aspects of life, and endless chatter in your head about them does the opposite of what hedonic motivation aims to achieve. The stream of thoughts pouring into your consciousness can not only produce persistent psychological pain but also cripple your cognitive capabilities.

Equanimity decouples you from your delusional thoughts or deceptive emotional feedback in the form of pain and pleasure, so that you can find peace and satisfaction in the absence of any real problem.

Even if you have real problem, delusions can make matters worse with ease. What you need is the cognitive clarity of an unshakable mind, so that you can use your executive functions to solve the problems of life, wrapped in complexities and ambiguities.

Equanimity prevents unnecessary suffering compelled by your own mind, freeing up your cognitive resources to be used to bring abundance into your life and make your life worthwhile.

Equanimity invokes courage and a challenge response, suppresses the fake fear and panic of a stress response, makes your nervous system work in a positive and powerful manner with the circuits of play and exploration, and enables you to face changes and challenges head on.

Some neuroscientific studies of decision-making suggest that many actions that appear to originate from your conscious free will are actually already initiated by unconscious neural activity in your brain, and some of this cognitive activity later leaks into your consciousness, giving you a sense of free will.

More research is needed to come to a conclusion on free will, but it is evident that thoughts are the result of conscious and unconscious activity, and free will is clearly not freely available to all, all the time. For example, quitting smoking or any other addiction, or feeling happy whenever you want, obviously need much more than a conscious, cognitive act of free will.

Thoughts, desires, and emotions can keep pouring into your consciousness, even when you want to shut them down just for a second. Cues from the environment can start a cascade of cognitive commotion that you wish you never had, and sometimes you feel bad without knowing why, because unconscious layers of awareness are beyond your reach.

The creation of your cognitions and emotions is not in your direct conscious control all the time, and self-control is never perfect, but it still works, and it is the only conscious cognition (and it becomes a cognitive skill with practice) that can save you from the tyranny of your self-activating cognitions and emotions.

The problems posed by your brain do not end with the delusions of hedonic motivation, and several known and unknown neural circuits are in place to make your life difficult; and yet you also possess the cognitive strength to control much of the conscious activity, provided there are no neurobiological deformities.

Self-control is the primary cognition that can control all other cognitions and emotions in your consciousness and your behaviors, and that can sculpt your subconscious brain in long run, one way or another, for your welfare. Sometimes mental and physical activities can be controlled in an instant, but you can also weed out unyielding, unadapting, and tenacious self-destructive learned behavior as you awaken your sleeping intellect and develop self-control over time.

Conscious cognitive control may be utterly difficult initially; however, as you get rid of the illusory emotions of hedonic motivation by equanimity and knowledge, you can slowly learn to control your mind.

Consciousness cannot be changed from its transient nature, and its contents cannot always be predefined. The self-executing survival software running in your head prefers negativity and unease to serenity and peace, even when the real difficulties of life give you a break.

Self-control stands between automatic thoughts and urges and subsequent emotions and actions, providing a cognitive delay whereby you can use your intellect to stop reacting to every cognition or emotion that infringes laws of sanity.

One cognitive skill is obviously not enough, and different cognitive strengths support each other. Self-control is likely to fail if you are dealing with the infinite illusions of desire and disgust. Knowledge of the extreme exaggerations of hedonic motivation, and being equanimous toward the dualities of pain and pleasure, can protect you from the real or fake feedback of emotions, and can give self-control room to operate.

An ability to control your focus helps you to fix your consciousness on problem-solving processes, which is certainly not an easy thing to do with a wandering mind. As you practice taking control of your attention with the use of detachment, self-awareness, and cognitive switching, self-control is also strengthened.

An action-focused life nullifies inbuilt mental and physical laziness, and along with life-supporting action, you also take action that gives purpose to your life; and you embark on a life-long journey that is beyond the dualities of pain and pleasure, stress and boredom, known and unknown, order and chaos, and the rest.

There are infinite ways to get lost in this world, and there are only a few ways to hold your ground no matter what. Subliminal systems in your brain can make your life difficult because of the irrational feedback of pain and pleasure, but at some level, they also seem to motivate you to do and become more.

The human brain deals with infinity using finite neural resources in a mind-boggling and incomprehensible manner, and imperfections are inevitable; but the brain is also equipped to deal with the finite—by allocating its limited neural resources to deal with a few goals.

The goals of survival and reproduction are most important, and plants do those things without any brain. The human brain is needed for survival in the social world, and for many, basic survival is still a huge challenge; however, not everyone in the world is happy when survival is not the current concern.

If you can aim at one long-term goal that defines the purpose of your life and it makes sense to you, you give your brain a much needed focal point to follow, and this changes everything for you. Your brain can never deal with infinite possibilities, but it can chase one realistic possibility; and no one knows what is realistic for the human brain. In the last millennium, which is a blink of an eye in the history of life, we have done what would have deemed impossible thousands of years ago.

Impossibility exists, obviously, but the fine line between the possible and the impossible is not always obvious.

By going after your purpose, you give your brain what it needs to function properly: one possibility, out of infinite possibilities. You can do things that seem impossible to you today; however, to do that you must focus your nervous system on one long-term possibility that also has a reason or meaning.

Perceptions are biased, and they are based on what you value and what motivates you. The world is largely unknown to a finite brain, and in general, you see what you want to see. A new world always awaits you in the unknown, which you can explore with a purpose and hope.

Finding a long-term goal is not an easy task, and you may need to first make sense of the world as it is. To understand where we are now, we need the wisdom and knowledge of our ancestors and fellow humans.

High-level knowledge of anthropology, archaeology, astronomy, biology, chemistry, economics, history (of the universe, life, and humans), intelligence (human and artificial), literature, neuroscience, philosophy, physics, politics, psychology, religion (for mythological or archetypal stories), sociology, and other relevant fields can help you to understand the sheer complexity of the universe and life.

Knowledge of complexity is of paramount importance to solve a complex problem, and dealing with the brain and the world, to suffer minimal and thrive, is a complex problem for most.

Knowledge can help you create a meaningful map of the world as you perceive it. Information is infinite, and not everything can be known. Being curious about the objective, mysterious universe is fine, but living with an eternal nihilistic and miserable confusion is not a great strategy for living life.

Along with knowledge, finding a purpose and pursuing it requires that you develop cognitive skills that make you smart and strong, and the skills which you develop in dealing with a long-term difficult goal makes the goal of mere survival extremely easy.

The acquisition of knowledge is needed. However, everything cannot be known, and every question cannot be answered. Having some humility about our limitations can keep the narcissistic human hubris and nihilism away.

No one knows what actual reality is. However, whatever helps you in your survival, and that of your family and community, with least amount of suffering, is the best definition of reality.

Most of the pain in the modern world is likely to be deceptive, and knowledge of illusions (of perceptions, cognitions, and emotions) can assist you to differentiate between real and fake.

You can never deal with the unrelenting illusory pain of arbitrary and transitory negative emotions that arise automatically from negativity bias, stress response, and other factors. You need to differentiate between the real and the unreal so that you can allocate your limited neural resources to cope with the real.

Without upfront knowledge of illusions, you will accept every false emotional alarm as the truth and suffer unnecessarily, in addition to compromising your ability to attend to authentic alarms. However, false alarms cannot be prevented all the time. Therefore, you need self-control, which can monitor the emotional contents of your consciousness for corrections in false feedback and direct your faculties of attention, cognition, and action toward solutions in the case of real feedback.

With equanimity and courage you endure both real and unreal pain patiently; a challenge response can regulate a stress response and related illusory emotions with confidence; and meditation supports the cognition of self-control to take control of your attention.

Purpose in your life assists self-control by allowing your motivation framework to focus on a finite goal and ultimately succeed, which can be done in most cases, whereas self-control is unlikely to do much productive work if there is no subjective moral hierarchy and you are lost in the infinity.

Pain is inevitable.

You do not know everything, you have not experienced everything, and you do not have every skill. As you move in space-time with your motivations, or are ruled by the laziness, you will always get emotional feedback. Sometimes it is unfair, sometimes it is needed for learning, and sometimes it is illusory.

However, you can alleviate and endure illusory or real pain with the help of cognitive fitness; and with it you can use your cognitive faculty to face the real challenges of life and thrive, using emotional pain as your guide. This is the original purpose of the pain, as long as there is something that you can do.

And in this way you can use pain to your advantage.

The experiences and philosophies of people are endless, and there is no single strategy that can work for everyone in every situation. Intellectual information, cognitive action, and clarity of mind may be needed if puzzling problems remain alive and misery has become a part of your life. Using cognitive action, you can solve the solvable problems of your life if you replace illusions with intellectual clarity, laziness with activity, and nihilism with meaning. This is the end goal of cognitive fitness.

ACKNOWLEDGEMENTS

This book is based on psychology and neuroscience; and you may also find a common theme of the Bible, Tao Te Ching, the Dhammapada, and the Bhagavad Gita. Thanks to all the scientists and philosophers, and our brave ancestors and fellow people.

The cover page and internal images are made using open-source software. Thanks to Inkscape (https://inkscape.org) and GIMP (https://www.gimp.org).

COGNITIVE YOGA

Yoga is popular around the world as meditation, breathing, and stretching exercises, and there is enough empirical evidence of its effectiveness. However, little is known about cognitive yoga, which focuses on exercising conscious cognitive control over motivation, cognition, action, and emotion.

Meditation, which is the yoga of focus (dhyana yoga, in Sanskrit) is the only form of cognitive yoga that is popular around the world; however, cognitive yoga focuses on the other elements of the mind and body as well.

Cognitive yoga is summarized nicely in the Bhagavad Gita, which is an ancient text written in the Sanskrit language and has around seven hundred verses; and it is also a part of the epic Mahabharata.

Some of the strategies discussed in this book have a resemblance to cognitive yoga from the Bhagavad Gita. For example, yoga of equanimity (sankhya yoga), yoga of action (karma yoga), yoga of self-control (atmasanyam yoga) and yoga of knowledge (gyan yoga).

Illusions and delusions are introduced in the Bhagavad Gita as maya and moha respectively. The purpose of your life is called dharma, and action is called karma.

Some verses of the Bhagavad Gita have a resemblance to counterintuitive quantum mechanics, some have huge psychological significance associated with them, and some are philosophical and spiritual.

It is hard to say why only meditation is popular and not the other forms of cognitive yoga, but one of the reasons is that other strategies suggested by the cognitive yoga seem paradoxical in nature.

But there is no other way.

Ambivalence and dissonance are inherent characteristics of your brain, and the brilliance of cognitive yoga is hidden in its puzzling paradox.

NOTES

INTRODUCTION

Müller-Lyer illusion: Müller-Lyer, FC (1889), "Optische Urteilstäuschungen"; Archiv für Physiologie Suppl. 263–270.

PAIN, PLEASURE, AND PURPOSE

Berridge, K.C. (2006). The debate over dopamine's role in reward: the case for incentive salience. Psychopharmacology, 191, 391-431.

Berridge, K.C., & Kringelbach, M.L. (2008). Affective neuroscience of pleasure: reward in humans and animals. Psychopharmacology, 199, 457-480.

Kringelbach, M.L. (2005). The human orbitofrontal cortex: linking reward to hedonic experience. Nature Reviews Neuroscience, 6, 691-702.

Panksepp, J. (1998). Affective Neuroscience: The Foundations of Human and Animal Emotions.

Parsons, C.E., Stark, E.A., Young, K.S., Stein, A.L., & Kringelbach, M.L. (2013). Understanding the human parental brain: a critical role of the orbitofrontal cortex. Social neuroscience, 8 6, 525-43.

Parsons, C.E., Young, K.S., Rochat, T.J., Kringelbach, M.L., & Stein, A.L. (2012). Postnatal depression and its effects on child development: a review of evidence from low- and middle-income countries. British medical bulletin, 101, 57-79.

INFORMATION AND ILLUSIONS

Café Wall illusion: Gregory, R.L. and Heard, P., 1979. Border locking and the Café Wall illusion. Perception, 8(4), pp.365-380.

Change blindness: O'Regan, J. K., Rensink, R. A., & Clark, J. L. Change-blindness as a result of "mudsplashes." Nature. doi:10.1038/17953; 1999. ; Davies G, Hine S. Change blindness and eyewitness testimony. The Journal of Psychology. 2007; 141(4): 423-434. ; Simons, D. J. & Rensink, R. A. Change blindness: Past, present, and future. Trends in Cognitive Sciences. 2005; 9(1): 16-20.

Close to 800 000 people die due to suicide every year. For every suicide there are many more people who attempt suicide every year: https://www.who.int/news-room/fact-sheets/detail/suicide

Inattentional blindness: Simons, D. J., & Chabris, C. F. (1999). Gorillas in our midst: Sustained inattentional blindness for dynamic events. Perception, 28, 1059-1074. ; Mack,

A., & Rock, I. (1998). MIT Press/Bradford Books series in cognitive psychology. Inattentional blindness. Cambridge, MA, US: The MIT Press.

Kahneman, D. (2003). Maps of Bounded Rationality: Psychology for Behavioral Economics.

Kahneman, D. (2011). Thinking, Fast and Slow.

Pohl, R.F. (2004). Cognitive illusions: A handbook on fallacies and biases in thinking, judgement and memory.

Simons, D.J., & Levin, D.T. (1998). Failure to detect changes to people during a real-world interaction. Psychonomic Bulletin & Review, 5, 644-649.

Tversky, A., & Kahneman, D. (1974). Judgment under Uncertainty: Heuristics and Biases. Science, 185 4157, 1124-31.

DUALITY, EQUANIMITY, AND COURAGE

Addis, D. R., Wong, A. T., & Schacter, D. L. (2007). Remembering the past and imagining the future: Common and distinct neural substrates during event construction and elaboration. Neuropsychologia, 45, 1363–1377.

Bernoulli, D. (1954). Exposition of a New Theory on the Measurement of Risk.

Berridge, K.C., & Kringelbach, M.L. (2008). Affective neuroscience of pleasure: reward in humans and animals. Psychopharmacology, 199, 457-480.

Berridge, K.C., & Robinson, T.E. (1998). What is the role of dopamine in reward: hedonic impact, reward learning, or incentive salience? Brain Research Reviews, 28, 309-369.

Berridge, K.C., Robinson, T.E., & Aldridge, J.W. (2009). Dissecting components of reward: 'liking', 'wanting', and learning. Current opinion in pharmacology, 9 1, 65-73.

Brickman, P., & Campbell, D.T. (1971). Hedonic relativism and planning the good society.

Duration neglect: Fredrickson, B. L., & Kahneman, D. (1993). Duration neglect in retrospective evaluations of affective episodes. Journal of Personality and Social Psychology, 65, 45-55.

Empathy gaps: Loewenstein, G, Prelec, D., & Shatto, C. (1998). Hot/cold intrapersonal empathy gaps and the under-prediction of curiosity. Unpublished manuscript, Carnegie Mellon University, Pittsburgh, PA. ; Loewenstein, G., & Adler, D. (1995). A bias in the prediction of tastes. The Economic Journal, 105, 929-937. ; MacDonald, T. K, MacDonald, G., Zanna, M. P., & Fong, G. T. (2000). Alcohol, sexual arousal, and intentions to use condoms in young men: Applying alcohol myopia to risky sexual behavior. Health Psychology, 19, 290-298. ; Loewenstein, G. (1996). Out of control: Visceral influences on behavior. Organizational Behavior and Human Decision Processes, 65, 272-292. ; Loewenstein, G. (2001). A visceral account of addiction. In P. Slovic (Ed.), Smoking: Risk, perception, & policy (pp. 188-215). Thousand Oaks, CA: Sage.

Gilbert, D.T. (2006). Stumbling on Happiness.

Helson, H. (1964). Adaptation-level theory: an experimental and systematic approach to behavior.

Illusion of unique invulnerability: Burger, J.M., & Burns, L. (1988). The Illusion of Unique Invulnerability and the Use of Effective Contraception. Personality & social psychology bulletin, 14 2, 264-270.

Immune neglect: Gilbert, D. T., Pinel, E. C, Wilson, T. D., Blumberg, S. J., &

Wheatley, T. P. (1998). Immune neglect: A source of durability bias in affective forecasting. Journal of Personality and Social Psychology, 75, 617-638.

Impact bias: Gilbert, D. T., Driver-Linn, E., & Wilson, T. D. (2002). The trouble with Vronsky: Impact bias in the forecasting of future affective states. In L. Feldman-Barrett & P. Salovey (Eds.), The wisdom of feeling (pp. 114-143). New York: Guilford. ; Larsen, R. J., & Fredrickson, B. L. (1999). Measurement issues in emotion research. In D. Kahneman, E. Diener, & N. Schwarz (Eds.), Well-being: The foundations of hedonic psychology (pp. 40-60). New York: Russell Sage Foundation. ; Hsee, C. K., & Abelson, R. P. (1991). Velocity relation: Satisfaction as a function of the first derivative of outcome over time. Journal of Personality and Social Psychology, 60, 341-347.

Kavanagh, D.J., Andrade, J., & May, J. (2005). Imaginary relish and exquisite torture: the elaborated intrusion theory of desire. Psychological review, 112 2, 446-67.

Kringelbach. M. L. (2009). The Pleasure Center: Trust Your Animal Instincts. New York: Oxford University Press.

Kringelbach. M. L., & Berridge, K. C (2010). Pleasures of the brain. New York: Oxford University Press.

Kringelbach. M. L., & Berridge, K. C. (2012). A joyful mind. Scientific American, 307, 40-45.

Kunda, Z. (1990). The case for motivated reasoning. Psychological bulletin, 108 3, 480-98.

Loewenstein, G., & Schkade, D.A. (1999). Wouldn't it be nice? Predicting future feelings.

Loss aversion: Kahneman, D. & Tversky, A. (1979). "Prospect Theory: An Analysis of Decision under Risk". Econometrica. 47 (4): 263–291. ; Kahneman, D. & Tversky, A. (1992). "Advances in prospect theory: Cumulative representation of uncertainty". Journal of Risk and Uncertainty. 5 (4): 297–323. CiteSeerX 10.1.1.320.8769. doi:10.1007/BF00122574.

Misconstrual problem: Griffin, D. W., & Ross, L. (1991). Subjective construal, social inference, and human misunderstanding. In M. Zanna. Advances in experimental social psychology (Vol. 24, pp. 319-356). New York: Academic Press. ; Milgram, S. (1974). Obedience to authority: An experimental view. New York: Harper & Row. ; Latane, B., & Darley, J. M. (1970). The unresponsive bystander: Why doesn't he help? Englewood Cliffs, NJ: Prentice Hall. ; Woodzicka, J. A., & LaFrance, M. (2001). Real versus imagined gender harassment. Journal of Social Issues, 57, 15-30.

Nearly 40% premature deaths in United States related to desire regulation: Schroeder, S. (2007) We Can Do Better Improving the Health of the American People. The New England Journal of Medicine, 357, 1221-1228.

O'Doherty, J., Kringelbach, M.L., Rolls, E.T., Hornak, J., & Andrews, C. (2001). Abstract reward and punishment representations in the human orbitofrontal cortex. Nature Neuroscience, 4, 95-102.

Okuda, J., Fujii, T., Ohtake, H., Tsukiura, T., Tanji, K., Suzuki, K., . . . Yamadori, A. (2003). Thinking of the future and the past: The roles of the frontal pole and the medial temporal lobes. NeuroImage, 19, 1369–1380.

Ordinization neglect: Wilson, Timothy D.; Daniel T. Gilbert (2003). Affective Forecasting. Advances in Experimental Social Psychology. 35. pp. 345–411. doi:10.1016/S0065-2601(03)01006-2. ISBN 9780120152353.

Pechmann, C., & Stewart, D.W. (2012). Advertising Repetition: A Critical Review of

Wearin and Wearout.

Peciña, S., & Berridge, K.C. (2005). Hedonic hot spot in nucleus accumbens shell: where do mu-opioids cause increased hedonic impact of sweetness? The Journal of neuroscience : the official journal of the Society for Neuroscience, 25 50, 11777-86.

Ratner, R.K., Kahn, B.E., & Kahneman, D. (1999). Choosing Less-Preferred Experiences for the Sake of Variety.

Robinson, T.E., & Berridge, K.C. (1993). The neural basis of drug craving: An incentive-sensitization theory of addiction. Brain Research Reviews, 18, 247-291.

Rolls, B.J., Rolls, E.T., Rowe, E.A., & Sweeney, K. (1981). Sensory specific satiety in man. Physiology & Behavior, 27, 137-142.

Schacter, D. L., Addis, D. R., & Buckner, R. L. (2008). Episodic simulation of future events: Concepts, data, and applications. Annals of the New York Academy of Sciences, 1124, 39–60.

Schacter, D. L., Addis, D. R., Hassabis, D., Martin, V. C., Spreng, R. N., & Szpunar, K. K. (2012). The future of memory: Remembering, imagining, and the brain. Neuron, 16, 582–583.

Suddendorf, T., & Corballis, M. C. (2007). The evolution of foresight: What is mental time travel and is it unique to humans? Behavioral and Brain Sciences, 30, 299–313.

Sunk cost fallacy: Mankiw, N. Gregory (2009). Principles of Microeconomics (5th ed.). Mason, OH: Cengage Learning. pp. 296–297. ISBN 978-1-111-80697-2.

Szpunar, K. K. (2010). Episodic future thought: An emerging concept. Perspectives on Psychological Science, 5, 142–162.

Tedeschi, R.G., & Calhoun, L.G. (1996). The Posttraumatic Growth Inventory: measuring the positive legacy of trauma. Journal of traumatic stress, 9 3, 455-71.

Tedeschi, R.G., & Calhoun, L.G. (2004). Posttraumatic Growth: Conceptual Foundations and Empirical Evidence.

Thompson, R.F., & Spencer, W.A. (1966). Habituation: a model phenomenon for the study of neuronal substrates of behavior. Psychological review, 73 1, 16-43.

SELF-CONTROL AND DETACHMENT

Aharon, I., Etcoff, N., Ariely, D., Chabris, C. F., O'Conner, E., & Breiter, H. C. (2001). Beautiful faces have variable reward value: fMRI and behavioral evidence. Neuron, 32, 537–551.

Ainslie, G. (1975). Specious reward: a behavioral theory of impulsiveness and impulse control. Psychological bulletin, 82 4, 463-96.

Anderson, M. C., Bjork, R. A., & Bjork, E. L. (1994). Remembering can cause forgetting: Retrieval dynamics in long-term memory. Journal of Experimental Psychology: Learning, Memory, and Cognition, 20, 1063–1087.

Anderson, R. C., Pichert, J. W., Goetz, E. T., Schallert, D. L., Stevens, K. V., & Trollip, S. R. (1976). Instantiation of general terms. Journal of Verbal Learning and Verbal Behavior, 15, 667–679.

Baddeley, A. D. (2001). Is working memory still working? American Psychologist, 56, 851–864.

Baddeley, A. D., & Hitch, G. J. (1974). Working memory. In S. Dornic (Ed.), Attention and performance (Vol. 6, pp. 647–667). Hillsdale, NJ: Erlbaum.

Bandura, A. (1965). Influence of models' reinforcement contingencies on the acquisition of imitative responses. Journal of Social and Personality Psychology, 1, 589–595.

Baumeister, R.F., & Heatherton, T.F. (1996). Self-Regulation Failure: An Overview.

Bayley, P. J., Frascino, J. C., & Squire, L. R. (2005). Robust habit learning in the absence of awareness and independent of the medial temporal lobe. Nature, 436, 550–553.

Bazerman, M.H., Tenbrunsel, A.E., & Wade-Benzoni, K.A. (1998). Negotiating with Yourself and Losing: Making Decisions with Competing Internal Preferences.

Beck, A. T. (2005). The current state of cognitive therapy: A 40-year retrospective. Archives of General Psychiatry, 62, 953–959.

Bekinschtein, T. A., Peeters, M., Shalom, D., & Sigman, M. (2011). Sea slugs, subliminal pictures, and vegetative state patients: Boundaries of consciousness in classical conditioning. Frontiers in Psychology, 2, article 337. doi:10.3389/fpsyg.2011.00337

Bloom, C. M., Venard, J., Harden, M., & Seetharaman, S. (2007). Non-contingent positive and negative reinforcement schedules of supersitious behaviors. Behavioural Process, 75, 8–13.

Bouton, M. E. (1988). Context and ambiguity in the extinction of emotional learning: Implications for exposure therapy. Behaviour Research and Therapy, 26, 137–149.

Bower, G. H. (1981). Mood and memory. American Psychologist, 36, 129–148.

Broberg, D. J., & Bernstein, I. L. (1987). Candy as a scapegoat in the prevention of food aversions in children receiving chemotherapy. Cancer, 60, 2344–2347.

Brown, S. C., & Craik, F. I. M. (2000). Encoding and retrieval of information. In E. Tulving & F. I. M. Craik (Eds.), The Oxford handbook of memory (pp. 93–107). New York: Oxford University Press.

Buchanan, T. W. (2007). Retrieval of emotional memories. Psychological Bulletin, 133, 761–779.

Carver, C.S., & Scheier, M.F. (1998). On the Self-Regulation of Behavior.

Casey, B.J., Jones, R.M., & Hare, T.A. (2008). The adolescent brain. Annals of the New York Academy of Sciences, 1124, 111-26.

Choy, Y., Fyer, A. J., & Lipsitz, J. D. (2007). Treatment of specific phobia in adults. Clinical Psychology Review, 27, 266–286.

Clark, R. E., & Squire, L. R. (1998). Classical conditioning and brain systems: The role of awareness. Science, 280, 77–81.

Clark, R. E., Manns, J. R., & Squire, L. R. (2002). Classical conditioning, awareness and brain systems. Trends in Cognitive Sciences, 6, 524–531.

Cognitive distortions: Beck, A. T. (1976). Cognitive therapies and emotional disorders. New York: New American Library. ; Burns, D. D. (2012). Feeling good: The new mood therapy. New York: New American Library. ; Leahy, R.L. (2017). Cognitive Therapy Techniques, Second Edition: A Practitioner's Guide. New York: Guilford Press. ; McKay, M. & Fanning, P. (2016). Self-Esteem: A Proven Program of Cognitive Techniques for Assessing, Improving, and Maintaining Your Self-Esteem. New York: New Harbinger Publications.

Cooper, J. C., Hollon, N. G., Wimmer, G. E., & Knutson, B. (2009). Available alternative incentives modulate anticipatory nucleus accumbens activation. Social Cognitive and Affective Neuroscience, 4, 409–416.

Delgado, M. R., Frank, R. H., & Phelps, E. A. (2005). Perceptions of moral character modulate the neural systems of reward during the trust game. Nature Neuroscience, 8, 1611–1618.

DeYoung, C.G., Quilty, L.C., & Peterson, J.B. (2007). Between facets and domains: 10 aspects of the Big Five. Journal of personality and social psychology, 93 5, 880-96.

Dickinson, A., Watt, A., & Griffiths, J. H. (1992). Free-operant acquisition with delayed reinforcement. Quarterly Journal of Experimental Psychology Section B: Comparative and Physiological Psychology, 45, 241–258.

Diffusion chain: Flynn, E., & Whiten, A. (2008). Cultural transmission of tool-use in young children: A diffusion chain study. Social Development, 17, 699–718.

Dillen, L.F., & Koole, S.L. (2007). Clearing the mind: a working memory model of distraction from negative mood. Emotion, 7 4, 715-23.

Domjan, M. (2005). Pavlovian conditioning: A functional perspective. Annual Review of Psychology, 56, 179–206.

Eich, J.E. (1980). The cue-dependent nature of state-dependent retention. Memory & Cognition, 8, 157–173.

Eich, J.E. (1995). Searching for mood dependent memory. Psychological Science, 6, 67–75.

Eichenbaum, H. (2008). Learning & memory. New York: Norton.

Eichenbaum, H., & Cohen, N. J. (2001). From conditioning to conscious recollection: Memory systems of the brain. New York: Oxford University Press.

Emmons, R.A. (1996). Striving and feeling: Personal goals and subjective well-being.

Evans, J.S. (2008). Dual-processing accounts of reasoning, judgment, and social cognition. Annual review of psychology, 59, 255-78.

Festinger, L. (1962). Cognitive dissonance. Scientific American, 207, 93-102.

Foa, E. B., Liebowitz, M. R., Kozak, M. J., Davies, S., Campeas, R., Franklin, M. E., . . . Tu, X. (2007). Randomized, placebo-controlled trial of exposure and ritual prevention, clomipramine, and their combination in the treatment of obsessive-compulsive disorder. Focus, 5, 368–380.

Gallistel, C. R. (2000). The replacement of general-purpose learning models with adaptively specialized learning modules. In M. S. Gazzaniga (Ed.), The new cognitive neurosciences (pp. 1179–1191). Cambridge, MA: MIT Press.

Garcia, J., & Koelling, R. A. (1966). Relation of cue to consequence in avoidance learning. Psychonomic Science, 4, 123–124.

Gershoff, E. T. (2002). Corporal punishment by parents and associated child behaviors and experiences: A meta-analytic and theoretical review. Psychological Bulletin, 128, 539–579.

Godden, D. R., & Baddeley, A. D. (1975). Context-dependent memory in two natural environments: On land and underwater. British Journal of Psychology, 66, 325–331.

Gottesman, I. I., & Hanson, D. R. (2005). Human development: Biological and genetic processes. Annual Review of Psychology, 56, 263–286.

Graf, P., & Schacter, D. L. (1985). Implicit and explicit memory for new associations in normal subjects and amnesic patients. Journal of Experimental Psychology: Learning, Memory, and Cognition, 11, 501–518.

Harreveld, F.V., Nohlen, H.U., & Schneider, I.K. (2015). The ABC of Ambivalence.

Harris, B. (1979). Whatever happened to Little Albert? American Psychologist, 34, 151–160.

Heatherton, T.F., & Wagner, D.D. (2011). Cognitive neuroscience of self-regulation failure. Trends in Cognitive Sciences, 15, 132-139.

Hoch, S.J., & Loewenstein, G. (1991). Time-inconsistent Preferences and Consumer Self-Control.

Hockley, W. E. (2008). The effects of environmental context on recognition memory and claims of remembering. Journal of Experimental Psychology: Learning, Memory, and Cognition, 34, 1412–1429.

Hofmann, W., Baumeister, R.F., Förster, G., & Vohs, K.D. (2012). Everyday temptations: an experience sampling study of desire, conflict, and self-control. Journal of personality and social psychology, 102 6, 1318-35.

Hofmann, W., Friese, M., & Strack, F. (2009). Impulse and Self-Control From a Dual-Systems Perspective. Perspectives on psychological science : a journal of the Association for Psychological Science, 4 2, 162-76.

Hofmann, W., Friese, M., Schmeichel, B.J., & Baddeley, A.D. (2011). Working memory and self-regulation.

Ideomotor effect: Shin, Y.K., Proctor, R.W., & Capaldi, E.J. (2010). A review of contemporary ideomotor theory. Psychological bulletin, 136 6, 943-74.

Jenkins, H. M., Barrera, F. J., Ireland, C., & Woodside, B. (1978). Signal-centered action patterns of dogs in appetitive classical conditioning. Learning and Motivation, 9, 272–296.

Kiefer, M., Schuch, S., Schenk, W., & Fiedler, K. (2007). Mood states modulate activity in semantic brain areas during emotional word encoding. Cerebral Cortex, 17, 1516–1530.

Knutson, B., Adams, C. M., Fong, G. W., & Hommer, D. (2001). Anticipation of increasing monetary reward selectively recruits nucleus accumbens. The Journal of Neuroscience, 21, 159.

Lattal, K. A. (2010). Delayed reinforcement of operant behavior. Journal of the Experimental Analysis of Behavior, 93, 129–139.

Lavine, H.G., Thomsen, C.J., Zanna, M.P., & Borgida, E. (1998). On the Primacy of Affect in the Determination of Attitudes and Behavior: The Moderating Role of Affective-Cognitive Ambivalence.

Loewenstein, G. (1996). Out of Control: Visceral Influences on Behavior.

May, J., Andrade, J., Kavanagh, D.J., Feeney, G.F., Gullo, M.J., Statham, D.J., Skorka-Brown, J., Connolly, J.M., Cassimatis, M., Young, R.M., & Connor, J.P. (2014). The craving experience questionnaire: a brief, theory-based measure of consummatory desire and craving. Addiction, 109 5, 728-35.

McGaugh, J. L. (2000). Memory: A century of consolidation. Science, 287, 248–251.

Mellon, R. C. (2009). Superstitious perception: Response-independent reinforcement and punishment as determinants of recurring eccentric interpretations. Behaviour Research and Therapy, 47, 868–875.

Metcalfe, J., & Mischel, W. (1999). A hot/cool-system analysis of delay of gratification: dynamics of willpower. Psychological review, 106 1, 3-19.

Milkman, K.L., Chugh, D., & Bazerman, M.H. (2009). How Can Decision Making Be Improved? Perspectives on psychological science : a journal of the Association for Psychological Science, 4 4, 379-83.

Mirror neurons: Rizzolatti, G., & Craighero, L. (2004). The mirror-neuron system. Annual Review of Neuroscience, 27, 169–192.

Moffitt, T. E. (2005). Genetic and environmental influences on antisocial behaviors: Evidence from behavioral-genetic research. Advances in Genetics, 55, 41–104.

Moffitt, T.E., Arseneault, L., Belsky, D.W., Dickson, N., Hancox, R.J., Harrington, H., Houts, R.M., Poulton, R., Roberts, B.W., Ross, S., Sears, M.R., Thomson, W.M., & Caspi, A. (2011). A gradient of childhood self-control predicts health, wealth, and public safety. Proceedings of the National Academy of Sciences of the United States of America, 108 7, 2693-8.

Mogenson, G.J., Jones, D.L., & Yim, C.Y. (1980). From motivation to action: Functional interface between the limbic system and the motor system. Progress in Neurobiology, 14, 69-97.

Morris, C. D., Bransford, J. D., & Franks, J. J. (1977). Levels of processing versus transfer-appropriate processing. Journal of Verbal Learning and Verbal Behavior, 16, 519–533.

Muraven, M., & Baumeister, R.F. (2000). Self-regulation and depletion of limited resources: does self-control resemble a muscle? Psychological bulletin, 126 2, 247-59.

Muraven, M., Tice, D.M., & Baumeister, R.F. (1998). Self-control as limited resource: regulatory depletion patterns. Journal of personality and social psychology, 74 3, 774-89.

Nairne, J. S., & Pandeirada, J. N. S. (2008). Adaptive memory: Remembering with a stone age brain. Current Directions in Psychological Science, 17, 239–243.

Ochsner, K.N., Ray, R.D., Cooper, J.C., Robertson, E.R., & Gross, J.J. (2004). For better or for worse: neural systems supporting the cognitive down- and up-regulation of negative emotion. NeuroImage, 23, 483-499.

Olsson, A., & Phelps, E. A. (2007). Social learning of fear. Nature Neuroscience, 10, 1095–1102.

Ono, K. (1987). Superstitious behavior in humans. Journal of the Experimental Analysis of Behavior, 47, 261–271.

Papies, E.K., Pronk, T.M., Keesman, M., & Barsalou, L.W. (2015). The benefits of simply observing: mindful attention modulates the link between motivation and behavior. Journal of personality and social psychology, 108 1, 148-70.

Pavlov, I. P. (1923). New researches on conditioned reflexes. Science, 58, 359–361.

Pavlov, I. P. (1923, July 23). Pavloff. Time, 1(21), 20–21.

Pavlov, I. P. (1927). Conditioned reflexes. Oxford, England: Oxford University Press.

Phelps, E. A., & LeDoux, J. L. (2005). Contributions of the amygdala to emotion processing: From animal models to human behavior. Neuron, 48, 175–187.

Povey, R.C., Wellens, B., & Conner, M.T. (2001). Attitudes towards following meat, vegetarian and vegan diets: an examination of the role of ambivalence. Appetite, 37, 15-26.

Rescorla, R. A., & Wagner, A. R. (1972). A theory of Pavlovian conditioning: Variations in effectiveness of reinforcement and nonreinforcement. In A. Black & W. F. Prokasky, Jr. (Eds.), Classical conditioning II (pp. 64–99). New York: Appleton-Century-Crofts.

Ridder, D.T., Lensvelt-Mulders, G., Finkenauer, C., Stok, F.M., & Baumeister, R.F. (2011). Taking stock of self-control: a meta-analysis of how trait self-control relates to a wide range of behaviors. Personality and social psychology review : an official journal of the Society for Personality and Social Psychology, Inc, 16 1, 76-99.

Roediger, H. L., III. (2000). Why retrieval is the key process to understanding human memory. In E. Tulving (Ed.), Memory, consciousness, and the brain: The Tallinn conference (pp. 52–75). Philadelphia: Psychology Press.

Rothbaum, B. O., & Schwartz, A. C. (2002). Exposure therapy for posttraumatic stress disorder. American Journal of Psychotherapy, 56, 59–75.

Rutter, M., & Silberg, J. (2002). Gene–environment interplay in relation to emotional and behavioral disturbance. Annual Review of Psychology, 53, 463–490.

Schacter, D. L. (2001). Forgotten ideas, neglected pioneers: Richard Semon and the story of memory. Philadelphia: Psychology Press.

Schacter, D. L. (2001). The seven sins of memory: How the mind forgets and remembers. Boston: Houghton Mifflin.

Schacter, D. L., & Tulving, E. (1994). Memory systems 1994. Cambridge, MA: MIT Press.

Sen, A. (1977). Rational Fools: A Critique of the Behavioral Foundations of Economic Theory.

Shefrin, H., & Thaler, R.H. (1977). An Economic Theory of Self-Control.

Sherry, D. F., & Schacter, D. L. (1987). The evolution of multiple memory systems. Psychological Review, 94, 439–454.

Skinner, B. F. (1938). The behavior of organisms: An experimental analysis. New York: Appleton-Century-Crofts.

Skinner, B. F. (1953). Science and human behavior. New York: Macmillan.

Skinner, B. F. (1972). The operational analysis of psychological terms. In B. F. Skinner, Cumulative record (3rd ed., pp. 370–384). New York: Appleton-Century-Crofts. (Original work published 1945.)

Sparks, P., Conner, M., James, R.J., Shepherd, R., & Povey, R. (2001). Ambivalence about health-related behaviours: an exploration in the domain of food choice. British journal of health psychology, 6 Pt 1, 53-68.

Squire, L. R., & Kandel, E. R. (1999). Memory: From mind to molecules. New York: Scientific American Library.

Stanovich, K.E., & West, R.F. (2000). Advancing the rationality debate.

Strotz, R.H. (1955). Myopia and inconsistency in dynamic utility maximization.

Tangney, J.P., Baumeister, R.F., & Boone, A.L. (2004). High self-control predicts good adjustment, less pathology, better grades, and interpersonal success. Journal of personality, 72 2, 271-324.

Thorndike, E. L. (1898). Animal intelligence: An experimental study of associative processes in animals. Psychological Review Monograph Supplements, 2, 4–160.

Tulving, E. (1972). Episodic and semantic memory. In E. Tulving & W. Donaldson (Eds.), Organization of memory (pp. 381–403). New York: Academic Press.

Tulving, E. (1983). Elements of episodic memory. Oxford, England: Clarendon Press.

Tulving, E. (1985). Memory and consciousness. Canadian Psychologist, 25, 1–12.

Tulving, E. (1998). Neurocognitive processes of human memory. In C. von Euler, I. Lundberg, & R. Llins (Eds.), Basic mechanisms in cognition and language (pp. 261–281). Amsterdam: Elsevier.

Tulving, E., & Schacter, D. L. (1990). Priming and human memory systems. Science, 247, 301–306.

Tulving, E., & Thompson, D. M. (1973). Encoding specificity and retrieval processes in episodic memory. Psychological Review, 80, 352–373.

Watanabe, S., Sakamoto, J., & Wakita, M. (1995). Pigeons' discrimination of painting by Monet and Picasso. Journal of the Experimental Analysis of Behavior, 63, 165–174.

Watson, J. B., & Rayner, R. (1920). Conditioned emotional reactions. Journal of Experimental Psychology, 3, 1–14.

Weissenborn, R. (2000). State-dependent effects of alcohol on explicit memory: The role of semantic associations. Psychopharmacology, 149, 98–106.

Wilcoxon, H. C., Dragoin, W. B., & Kral, P. A. (1971). Illnessinduced aversions in rats and quail: Relative salience of visual and gustatory cues. Science, 171, 826–828.

Winkielman, P., Berridge, K.C., & Wilbarger, J.L. (2005). Unconscious affective reactions to masked happy versus angry faces influence consumption behavior and judgments of value. Personality & social psychology bulletin, 31 1, 121-35.

Zhang, T. Y., & Meaney, M. J. (2010). Epigenetics and the environmental regulation of the genome and its function. Annual Review of Psychology, 61, 439–466.

ACT FOR A PURPOSE, NOT REWARDS

Ariely, D., Gneezy, U., Loewenstein, G., & Mazar, N. (2009). Large Stakes and Big Mistakes.

Fiorillo, C. D., Newsome, W. T., & Schultz, W. (2008). The temporal precision of reward prediction in dopamine neurons. Nature Neuroscience, 11, 966–973.

Fishbach, A., Friedman, R.S., & Kruglanski, A.W. (2003). Leading us not unto temptation: momentary allurements elicit overriding goal activation. Journal of personality and social psychology, 84 2, 296-309 .

Fredrickson, B.L. (1998). What Good Are Positive Emotions? Review of general psychology : journal of Division 1, of the American Psychological Association, 2 3, 300-319.

Fredrickson, B.L. (2001). The role of positive emotions in positive psychology. The broaden-and-build theory of positive emotions. The American psychologist, 56 3, 218-26.

Fredrickson, B.L., Mancuso, R., Branigan, C., & Tugade, M.M. (2000). The Undoing Effect of Positive Emotions. Motivation and Emotion, 24, 237-258.

Fujita, K., Trope, Y., Liberman, N., & Levin-Sagi, M. (2006). Construal levels and self-control. Journal of personality and social psychology, 90 3, 351-67.

Meule, A., Skirde, A.K., Freund, R.L., Vögele, C., & Kübler, A. (2012). High-calorie food-cues impair working memory performance in high and low food cravers. Appetite, 59, 264-269.

Papies, E.K., Potjes, I., Keesman, M., Schwinghammer, S., & Koningsbruggen, G.M. (2014). Using health primes to reduce unhealthy snack purchases among overweight consumers in a grocery store. International Journal of Obesity.

Rogers, T., & Bazerman, M.H. (2008). Future Lock-In: Future Implementation Increases Selection of 'Should' Choices.

Sweet, L.H., Mulligan, R.C., Finnerty, C., Jerskey, B.A., & Niaura, R.S. (2010). Effects of nicotine withdrawal on verbal working memory and associated brain response. Psychiatry Research: Neuroimaging, 183, 69-74.

Trope, Y., & Liberman, N. (2003). Temporal construal. Psychological review, 110 3, 403-21.

FOCUS AND MEDITATION

Epel, E.S., Daubenmier, J., Moskowitz, J.T., Folkman, S., & Blackburn, E.H. (2009). Can meditation slow rate of cellular aging? Cognitive stress, mindfulness, and telomeres. Annals of the New York Academy of Sciences, 1172, 34-53.

Goyal, M., Singh, S., Sibinga, E.M., Gould, N.F., Rowland-Seymour, A., Sharma, R., Berger, Z.D., Sleicher, D., Maron, D.D., Shihab, H.M., Ranasinghe, P.D., Linn, S., Saha,

S., Bass, E.B., & Haythornthwaite, J.A. (2014). Meditation programs for psychological stress and well-being: a systematic review and meta-analysis. JAMA internal medicine, 174 3, 357-68.

Hofmann, S.G., Sawyer, A.T., Witt, A.A., & Oh, D. (2010). The effect of mindfulness-based therapy on anxiety and depression: A meta-analytic review. Journal of consulting and clinical psychology, 78 2, 169-83.

Lazar, S.W., Kerr, C.E., Wasserman, R.H., Gray, J.R., Greve, D.N., Treadway, M.T., McGarvey, M.K., Quinn, B.T., Dusek, J.A., Benson, H., Rauch, S.L., Moore, C.I., & Fischl, B. (2005). Meditation experience is associated with increased cortical thickness. Neuroreport, 16 17, 1893-7.

Lutz, A., Slagter, H.A., Dunne, J.D., & Davidson, R.J. (2008). Attention regulation and monitoring in meditation. Trends in Cognitive Sciences, 12, 163-169.

Moore, A., & Malinowski, P. (2009). Meditation, mindfulness and cognitive flexibility. Consciousness and Cognition, 18, 176-186.

CONCLUSION

Burroughs, J.E., & Rindfleisch, A.P. (2002). Materialism and Well-Being: A Conflicting Values Perspective.

Clark, A.E., Frijters, P., & Shields, M.A. (2008). Relative Income, Happiness and Utility: An Explanation for the Easterlin Paradox and Other Puzzles.

Emmons, R.A. (1986). Personal strivings: An approach to personality and subjective well-being.

Gardner, J.P., & Oswald, A.J. (2007). Money and mental wellbeing: a longitudinal study of medium-sized lottery wins. Journal of health economics, 26 1, 49-60.

Gruber, J., Mauss, I.B., & Tamir, M. (2011). A Dark Side of Happiness? How, When, and Why Happiness Is Not Always Good. Perspectives on psychological science : a journal of the Association for Psychological Science, 6 3, 222-33.

Kahneman, D., Diener, E., & Schwarz, N.F. (1999). Well-being : the foundations of hedonic psychology.

Kasser, T. (2002). The High Price of Materialism.

Lucas, R.E., Clark, A.E., Georgellis, Y., & Diener, E.D. (2003). Reexamining adaptation and the set point model of happiness: reactions to changes in marital status. Journal of personality and social psychology, 84 3, 527-39.

Lyubomirsky, S., Sheldon, K.M., & Schkade, D.A. (2005). Pursuing Happiness: The Architecture of Sustainable Change.

Schwartz, B., Ward, A.T., Monterosso, J., Lyubomirsky, S., White, K., & Lehman, D.R. (2002). Maximizing versus satisficing: happiness is a matter of choice. Journal of personality and social psychology, 83 5, 1178-97.

Sheldon, K.M., & Kasser, T. (1998). Pursuing Personal Goals: Skills Enable Progress, but Not all Progress is Beneficial.

INDEX

Made in the USA
Coppell, TX
25 November 2020

42067948R00142